RIGHTS

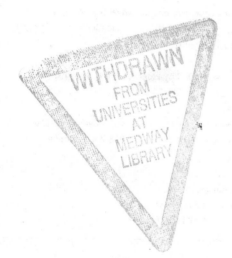

RIGHTS AND REALITIES

Comparing new developments in
long-term care for older people

Edited by Caroline Glendinning

The POLICY

P~P

PRESS

First published by in Great Britain in 1998 by

The Policy Press
University of Bristol
Rodney Lodge
Grange Road
Bristol BS8 4EA

Tele   +44 (0)117 973 8797
Fax   +44 (0)117 973 7308
e-mail   tpp@bristol.ac.uk
http://www.bristol.ac.uk/Publications/TPP

© The Policy Press, 1998

BWC

British Library Cataloguing in Publication Data

A catalogue record for this book is available from the British Library

ISBN 1 86134 125 3 (pbk)

Caroline Glendinning is Senior Research Fellow, National Primary Care Research and Development Centre, University of Manchester.

Front cover: Photograph supplied by kind permission of Mo Wilson, Format Photographers, London.

Cover design: Qube Design Associates, Bristol.

Printed and bound in Great Britain by Hobbs the Printers Ltd, Southampton.

Contents

List of tables and figures

Tables

Figures

Acknowledgements

We would like to express our grateful thanks to the many people who have helped with the writing and production of this book:

- Linda Hantrais and Alan Walker for support and encouragement to pursue the project beyond the early, doubtful stages.
- Jorma Sipila and Teppo Kroger, who read and commented on the draft of Chapter Five and Eeva Paivarinta for her extensive telephone advice.
- Lis Wagner, whose comments on earlier drafts enriched Chapter Six, especially in clarifying the role of experimental projects in wider policy formation and the historical sequence of events; Eigil Boll Hansen, who corrected factual errors and provided access to unpublished data; Myra Lewinter, who helped to locate Danish developments within an Anglo-Saxon perspective; Lis, Eigil, Myra, Elisabeth Toft Rasmussen and Merete Platz who gave up their time to discuss ideas in the early stage of the project and who provided valuable perspectives on the overall development of Danish policy for older people.
- Karen Turvey, Jenny Doyle, Cathy Thomson, Sheila Shaver, Peter Saunders and Lynn Sitsky (Social Policy Research Centre, University of New South Wales), Alan Owen, George Stathers, Brian Conway, Ros Sorensen, Don Hindle, Anna Howe and Ina Fine-Dekkers, for help with Chapter Seven.
- Margarita Cook, National Primary Care Research and Development Centre, University of Manchester, for invaluable work in transmitting drafts of chapters back and forth around the globe and putting together the final manuscript; other colleagues at NPCRDC for their patient tolerance of the pressures created by the writing and editing of the book; Fran Morris, for help with final copy-editing; Dawn Pudney, The Policy Press, for moral support and encouragement; and two referees who commented on an earlier draft.

The book grew out of a programme of research funded by the UK Department of Health at NPCRDC, University of Manchester, on the boundaries and interfaces between health and social welfare services. The views expressed in this book are those of the authors and not necessarily those of the NPCRDC or Department of Health.

Notes on contributors

Jan Coolen has a degree in sociology and economics and a PhD in public administration and public policy. He is currently a member of the Board of Directors of The Netherlands Institute of Care and Welfare and simultaneously Head of the Department of Social Care and Social Policy in the Institute. His main interests are in the transformation of the welfare state and social policy, structures of long-term care and innovation in health and social services.

Michael Fine BA(Hons), PhD, is Senior Research Fellow, Social Policy Research Centre, University of New South Wales, Australia, where he is currently involved in a number of evaluations of recent community care initiatives, including the NSW demonstration projects in community care and the coordinated care trial taking place in the north Sydney area. He is a member of the national executive of the Australian Association of Gerontology and a past president of the Australian Association of Gerontology (NSW Division).

Caroline Glendinning has degrees in sociology and social policy; she is currently Senior Research Fellow in the National Primary Care Research and Development Centre, University of Manchester, UK. She has conducted many studies of the implementation and impact of community care policies, including an earlier comparative study of financial support for family and informal care-giving. She currently leads a programme of research on the interfaces between primary health and social welfare services.

Kristiina Martimo BA(Soc), MA, lived in Finland for the first 24 years of her life and moved to England in 1975. She had BA and MA degrees in social policy from the University of Kent. She welcomed the opportunity to research and write the chapter on Finland, because her student life was based in England and this book gave her a deeper understanding of her country of origin.

Lone Lund Pedersen has a degree in political science (cand.scient.pol.). She is currently Research Associate in the National Primary Care Research and Development Centre, University of Manchester, UK. Here she is involved in two streams of work: 'interfaces between primary health and social services' and 'organisations, decision making and accountability in primary health care'.

Michaela Schunk recently received her doctorate from the University of Manchester, where she worked in the field of comparative research. She is currently Visiting Professor at the Institute for Health and Ageing, University of California at San Francisco.

Sylvia Weekers has a degree in health sciences, with policy and management being the main subjects. Her present position is researcher in the Department of Social Care and Social Policy at The Netherlands Institute of Care and Welfare. She has recently completed a study of home care and care allowances in the European Union.

ONE

Convergence or diversity in the provision of long-term care for frail older people?

Caroline Glendinning

Introduction

This book explores the changes which have taken place across a number of countries in the financing, scope and organisation of services and support for older people – typically those who, because of ill-health or frailty, need help with health, personal and/or social activities on a regular basis. The cornerstones of social policies and social welfare for older people – income security, minimum housing standards and access to health care (Hennessy, 1997) – are widely acknowledged to be unable to meet the expanding needs for long-term care. For example, in the UK a Royal Commission was established in late 1997 to explore the options for a sustainable system of funding long-term care for older (and younger disabled) people, including the appropriate balance between collective and individual financial responsibilities. Furthermore the traditional forms of social welfare provision are also considered inappropriate for long-term care needs; hospitals and other institutional settings, for example, are no longer considered desirable locations for long-term care.

However, it is simplistic to assume a straightforward, direct relationship between demographic pressures and changes in the funding, location, organisation or delivery of services. The formulation and implementation of policy is never so simple. Service responses to demographic trends such as these are also shaped by underlying global trends and ideologies which, on the one hand, tend towards convergent outcomes. On the other hand, developments in policies and services are also shaped by the histories, institutional and cultural traditions of individual welfare states; these individualised characteristics may, to a greater or lesser extent, place limits on the extent of any convergence.

Exploring these differences among a group of countries which are experiencing similar pressures is valuable for a number of reasons. It offers opportunities for 'natural experiments' – the comparison of different service configurations and their outcomes. It offers an empirical basis for forward projections and speculation – what might be the consequences for health and social welfare services if, for example, devolution and regionalisation in the UK profoundly alter the current relationships between local and national governments in the funding and planning of services? Overall, examining the experiences of other countries expands our awareness of the potential options to be explored – and the pitfalls to be avoided – in developing appropriate policies, both in the UK and elsewhere.

Demographic trends

All advanced post-industrial societies have for some time been experiencing major changes in their demographic profiles. Both the absolute numbers of older people and the proportions of total populations which they constitute are increasing; these increases will continue for the next four decades. By the year 2020, people aged 65 and over are expected to represent almost a fifth (18.6%) of the population of OECD (Organisation for Economic Cooperation and Development) countries, with very elderly people (75-plus) approaching one in ten of the total OECD population by 2025 (OHE, 1997, Tables 1.7 and 1.8). At least a substantial proportion of the new cohorts of younger retired people will enjoy good health and continue to make substantial contributions to voluntary and informal activities. However, the incidence of morbidity among older people tends to be two to three times higher than in the general population, with correspondingly higher levels of hospital use and sickness insurance claims (Walker and Maltby, 1997, p 92). It is the anticipated increase in the numbers of very elderly people (aged 80 and over), as the post-Second World War baby boom ages, which is expected to have a major impact on demand for health and social services.

These widespread demographic trends are being accompanied by corresponding decreases in birthrates. During the next 50 years the ratio of older, retired to working age people in the UK is expected almost to double, from 29 retired people per 100 of working age in 1994 to 43 per 100 in 2051 (ONS, 1997). Changes in the demographic balance between working age and retired people, in turn, raise questions about the levels of resources for funding welfare transfer payments and services which can be generated from a contracting economic base.

Whether or not these changes constitute a 'demographic timebomb' is a matter of some controversy (Tester, 1996; Hugman, 1996). Even among the very much older age groups, who are at greater risk of ill-health and infirmity, demands on health and other services are likely to vary considerably, partly reflecting life-long inequalities in living standards and personal resources. At any one time, those older people making significant use of health services constitute a minority (Estes, 1986). Although older people use health services more than other age groups, it is far from clear that these demographic trends "are the key to explaining rising health care expenditure" (Jamieson, 1989, p 446).

Nevertheless, these major demographic shifts have presented major challenges to the capacity of health and welfare services which were designed to provide for rather different population profiles. "The claims of older people to particular forms of health and welfare services have become highly contestable ..." (Hugman, 1996, p 212). In particular, they are prompting a rethinking of the boundaries between public and private responsibilities for funding and providing care – a shift which, in the UK at least, has arguably been characterised more by administrative stealth than by democratic debate and public legitimation. These demographic pressures are also prompting major renegotiations of the boundaries between, and within, the health and social welfare systems which are at the heart of most post-industrial welfare states.

Political and policy pressures

These demographic trends are being accompanied by widespread changes in both political ideologies and economic orthodoxies, which are radically altering traditional assumptions about the role of welfare states and welfare services. These trends are far from exclusive to the UK; rather, they provide a framework for the major social and economic restructuring which most 'western' welfare states are undergoing.

In the UK, economic constraints since the mid-1970s have placed increasing restrictions on the expansion of public expenditure and public services to meet changing needs and demands. From the mid-1970s, too, political ideologies have challenged conventional assumptions about the role of the welfare state in providing security 'from the cradle to the grave'. The traditional notion of state-provided welfare as a social right based on citizenship has been challenged; instead "there is increasing acceptance of the idea that the welfare state should do no more than guarantee a minimum level of support" (Henry Cox, 1998, p 13). Instead of single, vertically-structured service providers, welfare services are increasingly characterised by pluralism and diversity. The term 'welfare mix' has been coined to describe this change (Evers, 1993). The 'top-down', centralised planning and coordination of services is being replaced by devolved, local functions; the emphasis is increasingly on the coordination of 'flat' networks of providers rather than the articulation of vertical hierarchies.

These political developments have played a crucial part in shaping policy responses to the growing demands for long-term care services which have arisen from the demographic changes described above. A central component of the political and economic paradigms which have dominated developments over the past two decades has been the introduction of quasi-markets into welfare services. Instead of health and social welfare services being provided by a single, monopoly provider, encouragement has been given to the development of a range of alternative providers of services. 'Purchasers' – whether individuals or organisations – then choose which particular provider best meets their need. Quasi-markets fulfil two objectives, one economic and one political. Economically, they introduce opportunities for competition between service providers, in the expectation that this will end provider monopolies and thus drive down costs. Politically, they embody and promote values of increased freedom and choice, in the place of the passive and undiscerning receipt of services.

The changes in policy and practice which have resulted also frequently involve redefining and reorganising the traditional institutional, professional and funding boundaries and responsibilities which have hitherto provided the framework of modern welfare states. These include the boundaries between hospitals and community-based health services; between institutional and home-based care; between formal and informal providers of care; between cash transfer payments and services 'in kind'; between public and private sector providers; and between national, regional and local levels of government. To some extent these challenges to traditional boundaries also reflect policies of 'substitution' – the search for less costly, but equally effective, types of services and support.

The consequences of welfare reform for frail older people

The combination of demographic pressures, economic restraint and changing political orthodoxies has had a particularly marked impact on services for frail older people. According to Baldock and Evers (1991a), services for older people are in the 'front line' of social policy developments. Reviewing developments in three European countries, they argue that the acute pressures placed on conventional service arrangements have led to major changes in patterns of services for older people. These changes, they suggest, are indicative of changes that are likely to happen throughout welfare systems more generally. "Welfare systems change first at points of pressure where established policies and solutions are no longer working or cannot be sustained" (Baldock and Evers, 1992, p 289).

As a result, according to Baldock and Evers, frail older people are in the front line of trends away from "state-dominated post-war patterns of welfare service provision" towards more "diffuse and pluralistic forms of social care". Care is increasingly home-based rather than located in large institutions. Rather than being the responsibility of, at most, a few organisations which monopolise service provision, care is increasingly coordinated from a number of different sources. Baldock and Evers argue that this is part of a more general development in which welfare services are moving from a pattern of "bureaucratic centralism" to one which they term "regulated pluralism". This is evidenced in the shift from "monopolistic public provision to [a] pluralistic mix of welfare providers"; in the replacement of "fragmented services" by "coordinated systems of services"; and in the move away from "state responsibility for the dependent" towards a "division of responsibility between state, family and voluntary sectors" (Baldock and Evers, 1992, p 291).

However, although the pressures on post-industrial welfare states may be similar, their responses to these pressures and the consequent changes in the scope and organisation of services may be more diverse. A considerable amount of discussion and debate has taken place about the delineation of different 'typologies' or 'families' of welfare states (Esping Anderson, 1990; Castles, 1993). The differences which have been identified in the philosophies and institutions of the various welfare state models suggest that it may not be appropriate to assume there is a simple convergence among different countries towards a single model of services for frail older people. If groups of welfare states can be distinguished by their different principles, philosophies and institutional structures, then these distinctions will also shape and differentiate their responses to common demographic, economic and political pressures. The diverse traditions and institutions of different welfare states are therefore likely to exert as much influence over developments in services for frail older people as the more widespread demographic or economic imperatives[1].

It is exactly this tension between convergence and diversity which provides the rationale and the starting point for this book. Over the past 20 years in the UK, fundamental changes have taken place in both the funding and the organisation of services for frail older people. The taxation-funded National Health Service (NHS) has progressively withdrawn from providing convalescent and continuing nursing care for frail older people; policies of 'community care' have promoted long-term care in domiciliary rather than institutional settings; access to many publicly-funded care services is now severely restricted and subject to stringent income-testing; and residential and nursing home services (and, to a lesser extent, home care services) have been transferred from public to commercial and private sector provider organisations (Wistow, 1996). Close relatives are expected to play a major – and largely uncompensated and unsupported – role in providing support to frail older people. Indeed Wistow (1996, p 68) suggests that "something akin to an 'inverse care law' operates, by which those with access to informal carers are less likely to receive support from social services". Moreover, the range of activities which informal carers are called upon to perform increasingly extends well beyond providing social support and companionship, into intimate areas of personal care and even highly technical nursing care (Kirk and Glendinning, 1998).

These changes have implications for the social rights, citizenship and quality of life experienced by frail older people, as well as their families and others involved in providing support. Changes in arrangements for securing access to services and other forms of support – for example, a shift from universalistic NHS services to means-tested local authority services domains, or from social security entitlements to discretionary needs-testing – could have a major impact on levels of social exclusion. Within quasi-markets, older users of health and welfare services can be recast as 'consumers', giving an impression of greater choice and control. However, consumerism by no means equates with citizenship (Prior et al, 1995; Bynoe, 1996)[2]. Current and future cohorts of frail older people are likely to be increasingly differentiated by ethnic status (Atkin, 1998) and by income levels and capital assets (Falkingham, 1998). It may therefore be difficult for substantial subgroups of frail older people to take advantage of new opportunities for choice and control in a care market.

About this book

How have other countries, experiencing similar pressures and trends, responded? Is there evidence of widespread convergence, as Baldock and Evers imply? Do the different responses of other countries provide lessons and examples which can inform the development of policies and professional practice in the UK? This book explores these questions through case studies of policy changes and service developments in five other industrial and post-industrial societies: Germany, The Netherlands, Finland, Denmark and Australia.

Although comparative research in social policy is gradually extending beyond the study of social security systems to the organisation and allocation of services (for example, Baldock and Evers, 1991a; 1992; Evers et al, 1994; Alber, 1995, Anttonen and Sipilä, 1996), there is still little relatively little research which systematically examines a range of different services and cash allowances to explore the impact of changes and substitutions across and between them. This is not an easy task. Concepts and meanings differ across cultures; levels of services may be difficult to standardise; and the importance of different services may depend upon the context and circumstances in which they are delivered. For example, marked differences between countries in their levels of statutory home help services may need to be understood alongside variations in pensions and care allowances which allow older people in some countries to purchase substantial amounts of private domestic help.

Nevertheless, the development of comparative research into services is important because of the changing age profiles of post-industrial societies. It is access to different types of services, rather than income and earnings, which is likely to play a increasingly influential role in determining the quality of life of the growing proportions of these populations who are not active members of the labour market. Have other countries, for example, experienced increasing pressures on their hospital services and sought to move health services from hospital to community settings? To what extent have domiciliary and community-based services replaced long-term institutional care for frail older people? Have growing pressures for long-term care provision led to redefinitions of the responsibilities of health and social welfare services, or to redefinitions of public and private responsibilities for providing care? What mechanisms have been developed to ensure coordination between these community-based services and the specialist healthcare which many older people are also likely to need? To what extent have new choices been introduced between cash payments such as care allowance and services in kind? Have policies been introduced to shift the balance of responsibilities for funding and/or providing long-term care between collective and private domains?

This book examines these issues from the perspectives of a number of countries which have recently made changes to the organisation, funding or delivery of health and social welfare services for frail older people. Thus Germany has recently introduced a social insurance scheme to cover long-term care costs; both The Netherlands and Denmark are experimenting with new ways of coordinating services and, in particular, bridging the gap between home-based and institutional care for very frail older people; Finland has radically devolved responsibility for allocating resources and providing services entirely to local municipal levels; while Australia, with long traditions of a 'mixed economy' of nursing home and community services, is also experimenting with a wide range of incentives and organisational changes intended to increase cooperation and coordination across and between services.

However, these are more than simply descriptive studies. Alongside many of the organisational and funding changes, which are described in the book, have been changes in the means by which older people access and receive publicly-funded services. Assessment and care management, for example, are key mechanisms for coordinating, at a micro-level, services from a number of different sources. While undoubtedly important in ensuring that services are responsive to needs and effectively delivered, they also represent major strategies for cost containment, because they enable services to be 'targeted' at those who need them most. Thus, while older people may receive more individualised service 'packages', they may also experience a reduction in the social and citizenship rights which can accompany welfare universality. This book will therefore attempt wherever possible to link information on health and welfare service inputs with information on the outcomes for the beneficiaries of those services, and the impact on their social rights and citizenship.

Each chapter has been specially commissioned and written by authors familiar with the organisation of health and welfare services in each country. This has enabled the contributing authors to draw on original, own-language documentation, including research reports and other material which may be difficult to obtain overseas. Access to material such as this is particularly important in relation to evaluations which have been carried out of new policy initiatives or pilot experiments.

One of the difficulties in carrying out cross-national studies is that country-level comparisons may obscure very considerable variations in the levels and organisation of services *within* any particular country. The approach taken here allows such variations to be taken into account; indeed, they are of substantial interest in themselves, because of their potential impact on the equity of access to, and use of services by, older people. The final chapter will draw together the impact and consequences of these various developments for older citizens and on the lessons which can be learnt for the future development of health and social welfare provision in the UK.

Notes

[1] I am grateful to Michael Fine for this particular argument.
[2] I am grateful to Susan Pickard for this point.

TWO

Health and social care services for frail older people in the UK: changing responsibilities and new developments

Caroline Glendinning

Introduction

Until 1983, most of the formal care services received by older people in the UK were both publicly funded and provided directly by public sector organisations – the National Health Service (NHS) for acute hospital care, primary and community health services and long-stay nursing care; local authority social services departments for residential, home help and day care services; and housing departments for 'sheltered', warden–assisted accommodation. Despite the importance of coordination between these various services for older people with complex social and health problems, local authority and NHS services have retained almost intact their separate funding streams and managerial and accountability structures which were established in the late 1940s.

This chapter describes the major changes which have taken place since the early 1980s in the funding and organisation of health and social welfare services for frail older people in the UK. These changes have resulted from a number of different policy trends and imperatives. First, there has been a major reduction in the scope of long-term care services provided by the taxation-funded NHS and a shift in responsibility to more discretionary service domains, supplemented by increasing levels of individual financial contributions. Secondly, policies have sought to develop more home-based alternatives to institutional care although, as the chapter will argue, evidence of the success of these policies is at best equivocal.

Thirdly, from the late 1980s, welfare services for older people have been increasingly affected by the 'marketisation' of the welfare state. An internal market was introduced into the NHS in 1990 and, of particular importance to older people, a major new private sector market of residential homes, nursing homes and, to a lesser extent, domiciliary care providers has developed since the mid-1980s. All these developments have taken place within a context of continuing tight constraints on public expenditure, the introduction of cash-limited budgets and the consequent targeting of services on the most dependent and frail older people.

The chapter will argue that, on the whole, these various trends have not resulted in coherent, integrated policies for the provision of health and social care services for frail older people; despite many local pilot projects and service initiatives, services for many older people remain fragmented and poorly coordinated. Moreover, despite the rhetoric of consumerism in public services, many older people have little choice over the services available to them. Finally, neither the roles and responsibilities of collectively funded versus privately purchased welfare, nor the respective responsibilities of the state versus the family have been openly debated. The chapter concludes with a brief summary of some of the opportunities which are likely to arise in the future for addressing some of these issues through associated policy and service developments.

The changing boundaries of NHS care

NHS services, whether provided in hospital or the community, remain funded from general taxation and are by and large free at the point of delivery. However, the scope of these services, particularly for frail older people, has altered dramatically over the past 15 years. Both the scope and the volume of hospital in-patient services has been markedly curtailed in two major respects. First, there has been a major decline in the volume of long-term hospital provision for older people. Between 1980 and 1994, long-term care beds for older non-psychiatric patients in hospitals and other NHS facilities decreased by one third, from 55,600 to 37,500 (comparable data was not available on NHS places for people with mental health problems [HC, 1995]). This was during a period when the numbers of people aged 75 to 84 increased by 18% and the numbers aged 85-plus increased by 80% – the very groups likely to make the biggest demands on health and social services (OPCS, 1995).

Secondly, the average length of hospital stay for older people who are acutely ill or require surgery has been reduced. Technological developments such as day case and non-invasive surgery have facilitated marked reductions in the length of in-patient stay. These advances have combined with resource-related pressures to increase hospital efficiency and maximise the throughput of patients. Consequently patients of all ages are now discharged much earlier after illness or surgery, with convalescence and rehabilitation increasingly taking place outside the hospital ward. The average length of stay in hospital wards for older people almost halved between 1979 and 1986, from 77.5 days to 44.8 days (Walker, 1995). Within specialist geriatric hospital services, the average length of stay also fell, from 36 to 20 days between 1989/90 and 1994/95. In total, between 1983 and 1996 there was a 38% reduction in NHS acute and long-stay beds for older people (Audit Commission, 1997). "In effect, the NHS has increasingly narrowed its role to that of a provider of acute care" (Audit Commission, 1997, p 13).

In 1995, an attempt was made to halt further attrition of the boundaries of NHS services, when the Department of Health (DoH) issued a requirement that health authorities must review local needs for, and provision of, long-term healthcare services. The services to be reviewed included specialist medical and nursing care in hospital and the community, rehabilitation and convalescence services, palliative healthcare, respite care and specialist transport. Where the boundary was considered to have moved too far, health authorities were required to reinvest in NHS services (DoH, 1995). However, no national guidelines were given about what was an acceptable level of long-term care services; it was left to individual health authorities to judge whether or not the NHS services in their area were adequate. The House of Commons Health Committee noted with concern the risk that local guidelines on the boundaries between NHS and 'social care' services would create and reinforce substantial variations between different health authority areas in access to NHS services. Indeed, a survey of draft local guidelines concluded that: "We now have a large number of draft eligibility criteria ... concealing widely differing access to [NHS] continuing care beds and widely varying levels of continuing care provision" (Saper and Laing, 1995, p 2).

Moreover, relatively few additional resources were made available to reinvest in NHS long-term care services – £20m in 1996/97 and £25m in 1997/98, the latter being available only if it was matched by funding from local health authority budgets. These additional resources were in the form of 'Challenge Fund' monies, for which bids had to be made for specific local developments. Any other resources had to be found from existing budgets (Audit Commission, 1997).

The consequences of NHS disinvestment in long-term care

The reduction in the scope and volume of NHS services was facilitated by changes in social assistance regulations which, between 1983 and 1993, allowed poorer older people to claim the full costs (both 'hotel' and 'care') of a private residential or nursing home place from social security funding, solely on the basis of a test of financial means. This alternative source of funding enabled hospitals to reduce their levels of 'in-house' long-term and convalescence services and local authorities also disinvested in their own directly provided residential care services. The discharge of older patients from NHS hospitals to private sector nursing homes for convalescence, rehabilitation and long-term nursing and personal care became increasingly common. For example, in one region of England almost half of all admissions to private nursing homes in 1995/96 were of people who had been discharged directly from hospital (NWECP, 1996).

As a 'safety net' benefit, social assistance expenditure on long-term residential and nursing home care was not cash-limited but entirely demand-led. Social assistance expenditure on nursing home and residential care therefore increased exponentially, from £39m in 1982 to £2,530m in 1992 (Laing, 1993). This was reflected in a rapid expansion of the private residential and nursing home market throughout the 1980s, with a 242% increase in the number of private sector nursing and residential home beds between 1983 and 1996 (Audit Commission, 1997). However, there was no comparable source of demand-led public funding to stimulate the development of additional domiciliary and day care services, which might have provided increased or more flexible support to enable older people to remain in their own homes. Indeed, it has been argued that the ready availability of funding for institutional, but not domiciliary, services caused considerable 'upward substitution' – the use of more expensive or intensive services than were actually needed, because those which would be appropriate were not available. This was particularly marked among younger – and arguably less frail – older people; while the population aged 65-74 declined by 9% between 1979 and 1989, private institutional places for this age group actually increased by 15% (Walker, 1994).

It should not be inferred that these changes were necessarily to be deplored. Both historical and contemporary studies have been highly critical of the quality of life available to older people in long-stay institutional care (Townsend, 1963; Meacher, 1972; Clarke and Bowling, 1990). There were therefore some sound reasons for welcoming the closure of traditional large, long-stay institutional facilities. However, this disinvestment in hospital facilities for older people was not part of a coherent policy of shifting investment into community-based services to enable older people to remain living at home for as long as possible. Instead, "the political will to achieve hospital closures came chiefly from the desire to reduce public expenditure ... [which] resulted in people being relocated without adequate preparation" (Walker, 1994, p 7).

Another consequence of the reduction in NHS long-term care services was a growing shortfall in rehabilitation services to encourage the reacquisition of independence which has been impaired by illness or injury. Most rehabilitation services are still provided in hospital, despite the decreased role of the hospital in the post-acute and long-term care of older people. A recent literature review found a decline in opportunities for rehabilitation over the last decade, with shortfalls disproportionately affecting older people with long-term illnesses and disabilities. Rehabilitation services in community settings are still underdeveloped (Robinson and Turnock, 1998).

A third consequence has been the transfer of responsibilities for funding and providing long-term care services for older people from a universalist service free at the point of delivery – albeit dominated by professional medical and nursing judgements of need – to the more selective, residual and discretionary domain of local authority social welfare services, in which bureaucratic and procedural processes can now exert considerable influence over access to and levels of service provision (Ellis, 1995). Salter (1994) has characterised this as a move from the comprehensive, universal rights to healthcare which were associated with the establishment of the NHS in 1946, into the ill-defined and highly contingent domain of social rights. This move was finally completed through the implementation in 1993 of major changes in funding arrangements for 'community care' services.

The 1993 community care changes and their consequences

Needs for medical and nursing care or surveillance were not included in the assessment of eligibility for social assistance payments for nursing or residential home services during the 1980s. This led to increasing concern that older people with lower levels of dependency were choosing to enter residential care at least partly because of the absence of appropriate home-based alternatives (Bradshaw and Gibbs, 1988). Social assistance payments were considered to provide a 'perverse incentive' to seek institutional care which contradicted official policies of 'community care'. In 1993, changes were therefore introduced to curb access to social assistance payments for private nursing home and residential services. Responsibility for both managing overall public spending on residential and nursing home care and for assessing potential applicants was transferred from the national social security system to local authority social services departments. Assessments now had to consider not only the financial circumstances but also the functional needs and social circumstances of older people. The transfer of resources for residential and nursing home placements to local authority social services departments created a single budget for both institutional and domiciliary care services; it was hoped that this would facilitate greater budgetary flexibility and create opportunities to switch investment into lower cost home and day care services.

Research on the implementation of the 1993 changes concluded that their "deep normative core" of curbing expenditure on long-term care had succeeded, through the transfer of a carefully calculated sum from the social assistance to local authority social services budget; and by making social services departments responsible for rationing expenditure on both residential and domiciliary care services (Lewis and Glennerster, 1996). Because of the earlier changes in acute and long-term NHS services for older people, the 'social' care responsibilities which local authority social services departments took on in 1993 included many aspects of long-term care which had previously been defined as 'health' needs, particularly convalescence and long-term nursing care.

Developing a 'mixed economy' of welfare

The 1993 'community care' changes also provided an opportunity to affirm a new role for local authority social services departments, as planners and purchasers rather than direct providers of services. Indeed, many local authorities had already ceased to provide their own residential care services and had transferred the ownership and management of former local authority accommodation to independent, not-for-profit trusts. However, the growth in the private residential and nursing home market during the 1980s had been largely opportunistic and highly variable across the country (Corden, 1992); local authorities were now charged with responsibility for managing that market. The shift was analogous to the 'purchasing' role of the new health authorities which had been created with the introduction of the NHS internal market in 1990 (Lewis and Glennerster, 1996, p 12).

There was particular concern that the transfer of resources from the social security budget to local authorities and its capping would destabilise the now substantial independent residential and nursing home sector. This would have been unfortunate for a government which, at the time, had a very strong commitment to reducing monopoly supply by local authorities and increasing choice for service users. Consequently the transferred funding was accompanied by a requirement that 85% of it must be spent on the purchase of non-local authority services. It is clear, however, that a policy of maintaining stability within the private residential and nursing home market is not entirely compatible with the development of services to enable very frail older people to remain in their own homes, as might be implied by the term 'community care'.

In addition to maintaining stability in the private residential and nursing home sector, the requirement that 85% of the transferred social security funding was to be spent on non-local authority services was also intended to stimulate the growth of independent providers of day and domiciliary care services. Provision of these services by the private sector was relatively underdeveloped and hitherto used mainly by people who could pay for services themselves; there had been no financial incentives to stimulate the supply of private domiciliary care services comparable to that offered to private institutional care providers by the social security payments of the 1980s (Perkins and Allen, 1997).

However, the development of day care and home care services by independent sector providers has been slow. There are substantial financial risks and difficulties in developing these services. Capital investment in a new domiciliary care service may be difficult to obtain without the security of the large premises which owners of nursing and residential homes can offer to lenders. It is difficult to combine the provision of flexible and responsive services, particularly at night and weekends when local authority home care services are usually not available, with the retention of a trained, reliable workforce which can provide the quality and continuity of care which are very important to older service users.

> **Balancing supply and demand, and keeping it balanced, is a continuing problem. Even when [fully] paid staff are employed, the greatest difficulty may lie not so much in recruiting them as in keeping them, especially if salaries are low or if the contract, and funding, is short-term or insecure. (Leat, 1993, p 31)**

Consequently, since 1993 considerable effort has gone into developing the capacity and expertise of local authority social services departments to stimulate and manage relationships with a range of non-statutory domiciliary service providers. The DoH-funded *Caring for people who live at home* initiative aimed to stimulate the development of both domiciliary and day care services by commercial and voluntary sector provider organisations; a wide range of innovative projects were developed in the 15 local authorities which took part.

The initiative highlighted the tensions between the encouragement of innovation and risk on the one hand and longer-term sustainability on the other: "the incompatibility of these two aims was never resolved" (Perkins and Allen, 1997, p 2). Subsequent monitoring and evaluation of the development of social care markets has found increasing maturity in the relationships between local authority purchasers and independent sector providers (Wistow et al, 1996). However, there may be trade-offs between the development of a diverse market in social care services on the one hand, and users' preferences on the other. A recent survey of over 1,000 older people found strong support for local authority home care services; only 16% of respondents said they would most trust private home care providers (Sykes and Leather, 1997). Other trade-offs are likely between flexibility and responsiveness and the market stability which can guarantee the continuity which older people value highly in home care services (Henwood et al, 1998). Consequently, four years after the 'community care' changes, there were still considerable restrictions on the range of domiciliary care providers which older service users could chose between. Two thirds of local authorities required priority to be given to their own, in-house services. Independent providers tended to be used only when in-house services were not available (for example, at evenings and weekends) or where difficulties had previously arisen in relationships between in-house providers and service users (Audit Commission, 1997, p 32). The maximisation of consumer choice which is intended by the development of social care markets remains circumscribed, at least for older people who access home care services through their local social services department.

The role of assessment and care management

At a micro-purchasing level, the 1993 changes placed great emphasis on assessment and care management as the main methods of improving the targeting and coordination of services for individual older people. Assessment was intended to promote a needs-led, rather than service-driven, approach; care management was intended to maximise the appropriate tailoring of individualised 'packages' of services to the assessed needs and choices of the older person. However, because of stringent financial constraints on local authorities' budgets, assessment has increasingly been used as a mechanism for prioritising needs and restricting access to services for all but the most at risk (Davis et al, 1997). Indeed, many social services departments now ration access to assessment itself, through a range of managerial and bureaucratic procedures which effectively delay or circumvent the assessment process for all but those older people at the highest risk of harm (Rummery and Glendinning, 1997b).

Care management was intended to allow the construction of flexible, coordinated 'packages' of services, in response to individual needs. Although local authority social services departments have lead responsibility, assessment and care management functions can be delegated to other professionals and organisations – particularly primary and community health services (DoH/SSI/Scottish Office SWSG, 1991a; 1991b). Guidance issued before the 1993 changes urged local authority and NHS organisations to develop collaborative care management and assessment procedures between them so that, for example, professionals could not only collect information for assessment purposes on each other's behalf, but also "be trusted to interpret that information and to access the resources of the other agency without further assessment" (DoH/SSI/Scottish Office SWSG, 1991a, p 89).

Care management may work well in relation to the purchasing and coordination of services which are funded by the care manager's own organisation. However, care managers have generally been far less successful in exerting leverage over and coordinating services which are funded by other organisations; which are provided by other professionals with their own management and accountability structures; and which are also likely to have their own assessment and eligibility criteria. For example, older people who need both home nursing and home care services may have to undergo separate assessments by both local authority social services staff and NHS community nursing staff, because the social services care manager has no means of purchasing nursing services (Glendinning, 1994). Multi-disciplinary teams in which social workers can carry out assessments for home nursing and nurses carry out assessments for home care services are by no means common (Rummery and Glendinning, 1997a). More recently, the Audit Commission has also pointed to the problems of poor coordination between professionals, leading to the risk of "either no assessment or 'serial assessment' by a myriad of professionals" (Audit Commission, 1997, p 24). The separate funding streams, management and accountability structures of local authority and NHS services impose very considerable barriers to joint working at all levels and do not lend themselves easily to marginal transfers of responsibility and funding in the light of local agreements and arrangement (Audit Commission, 1992). For both NHS and social services organisations concerned about reconciling rising demands with limited budgets, there is "no incentive, and potentially large penalties, for such common law marriages" (Salter, 1994, p 128).

The development of charging policies for community care services

Under the new 'community care' arrangements, a considerable tranche of long-term care services previously provided free of charge by the NHS are now subject to financial charges to users, the level depending on their financial circumstances. Entrants to residential or nursing homes are now required to contribute to the costs, depending on their income and assets. Those with assets over £10,000 (including the value of a home or other property) must make a financial contribution; those with assets over £16,000 must pay the full cost. Regulations inherited from the pre-1993 social security funding regime deter older people from 'spending down' or transferring assets to relatives in anticipation of a possible admission to institutional care. Controversially, because of the 1980s' changes in NHS services and the availability of social security funding, coupled with the 1993 'community care' changes, these charges now cover all personal and nursing care which is provided in institutional settings.

Moreover, since the early 1980s, the majority of local authorities have introduced, and subsequently increased, charges or co-payments for home help and day care services; only the poorest older people are likely to be exempt (NCC, 1995; Chetwynd et al, 1996). Although the 1993 'community care' changes introduced a single, national means test to determine the level of an older person's contribution to the costs of institutional care, charges for home care and day care services are left to the discretion of individual local authorities. Consequently, the contributions expected from older people can vary considerably, both between local authorities and between different services and 'client groups' *within* any single local authority. Many older people therefore anticipate increases in their care needs with considerable anxiety, as the lack of consistency in financial assessment and charging policies makes it difficult for them to predict the financial implications of increased service inputs (Baldwin and Lunt, 1996).

The consequences of the community care changes for older people

The withdrawal of the NHS from the provision of long-term nursing and rehabilitation services and the 'community care' changes in 1993 have together had a number of consequences for the range of publicly funded services for older people and the conditions under which these services are obtained.

The shift from public to private responsibilities

First, there has been an overall shift in responsibilities for the funding of long-term care services from the NHS to individual older people and their families. Although the medical and nursing services provided by family doctors and community nurses for older people living in their own homes are still funded from general taxation and free at the point of delivery, nursing and personal care provided in institutional settings is not. The availability of social security funding between 1983 and 1993 masked a major withdrawal by the NHS from this area of responsibility. When the availability of social security funding ended in 1993, the new financial assessments introduced by local authorities enabled them to levy substantial financial contributions, not just from entrants to residential care homes but from older people entering nursing home care as well. These charges also apply to older people who might use nursing or residential homes on a short-term basis, for example, for respite or convalescence. The introduction and extension of charges for local authority home care and day care services has increased yet further the financial contributions expected of older people towards the costs of their long-term care services.

These changes have not been openly debated. Older people now find themselves charged for services which they had expected to be provided free in return for the contributions which they had made through taxation and national insurance during their working lives (Joseph Rowntree Foundation, 1996; Diba, 1996). Disquiet has also been expressed about the greatly increased risk that the value of their home, which older people had expected to bequeath to their families, will have to be spent on the costs of institutional care. This anxiety should be placed within the context of policies which have actively encouraged the extension of home ownership – now the most common source of capital asset in the UK – and the creation and inheritance of personal wealth (Hamnett, 1995). A number of schemes have been proposed to resolve this funding problem

(Laing, 1993; Harding et al, 1996; Richards et al, 1996; Joseph Rowntree Foundation, 1996; HMSO, 1997). In 1997 a Royal Commission on long-term care was appointed to consider future policy in this area; hopefully its recommendations, due to be published early in 1999, will provide a basis for much needed public consultation and discussion about the balance of public and private responsibilities.

Partly because of the increased 'targeting' of services by local authorities on older people who are most at risk, many older people rely very heavily on the help and support of friends and close relatives in order to stay in their own homes for as long as possible. This informal help is given not only for domestic and household tasks but also for personal care and, increasingly, for tasks which were previously the domain of professional nurses (Kirk and Glendinning, 1998). The value of the help given to older and younger disabled people by informal carers was estimated to have reached £39.1 billion in 1992 (Laing, 1993). Although the UK is unusual, compared with some other EU countries, in having a social security benefit specifically for people providing substantial amounts of informal care to a disabled or older person, the benefit is only payable to carers of working age. It is therefore received by a relatively low proportion of the target population. Moreover, it is much lower than care allowances in other countries, which also go directly to the older people themselves so that they can exert a degree of influence over how and to whom they should be paid (Glendinning and McLaughlin, 1993a).

The failure of 'community care'

Despite the 1993 changes, there is evidence that domiciliary and day care services remain far from adequate. This is manifest in a number of ways. First there are concerns that older people not in need of medical care may be admitted to hospital simply for want of alternative arrangements. Although only an imprecise indicator, between 1982 and 1994 the proportions of the over-75 age group admitted to hospital increased from 13 to 18% (Audit Commission, 1997). There is, however, clear evidence that increasing levels of home care services are being concentrated on smaller numbers of high risk clients (LGMB, 1997). This suggests that opportunities for earlier, preventative service interventions may be overlooked in the pressure to target services on those most at risk. Moreover, when a crisis does occur, it may be difficult to put domiciliary services in place or find residential accommodation sufficiently quickly. The financial pressures on social services departments make it difficult for them to fund purely preventive services. Indeed, in some areas these pressures are so severe that the number of places in residential nursing homes has had to be limited; new applicants are therefore likely to be placed on a waiting list (Audit Commission, 1997).

Thirdly, admissions to long-stay nursing and residential care homes remain high. In 1995/96, 64% of English local authorities' gross expenditure on services for people aged 75-plus was on care in residential settings (Audit Commission, 1997, p 34). Between March 1993 and March 1996, the number of residents supported financially by local authorities in nursing and residential homes increased by 112% (LGMB, 1997). In the following year, to March 1997, the numbers increased by a further 12% (DoH, 1997a). This partly reflects the slow and patchy development, described above, of a mixed economy of flexible, responsive, domiciliary and community-based services; "a ready supply of residential and nursing homes was at hand while independent sector home care was relatively underdeveloped" (Audit Commission, 1997, p 47). It also reflects the introduction of a new 'perverse financial incentive' into charging frameworks for local authority services; the capital available from the sale of an older person's home can be taken into account in assessing their contribution towards the costs of institutional care but not the costs of home care services where user charges are based on income alone. It is therefore usually substantially cheaper for local authorities to place people in institutional care, even where there is no difference in the gross costs of institutional and domiciliary services (Audit Commission, 1996).

Local variations in community care services

Whether or not major variations existed before 1983 in the services available to frail older people in different areas is not clear. Certainly, professional (particularly medical) judgements would have exerted considerable influence over whether long-term hospital and other medical services were provided.

However, it is arguable that the policy shifts of the 1980s and 1990s have both increased variations between different areas and made them more visible. The influence of welfare mix and marketisation policies has led to the very uneven development of both institutional and domiciliary services. The lack of national guidelines on eligibility for continuing NHS care has meant further variations in the boundaries between 'health' and 'social' care services. Local authorities themselves inherited very different service patterns and priorities in 1993. As a result, very wide variations – from 20 to 70% – are apparent in the proportions of people referred for community care services who subsequently receive a full assessment; in the maximum amounts which local authorities are willing to spend on domiciliary services for individual users; and in average levels of home care and home help services provided to individual households (Audit Commission, 1996). "The result of this fragmentary innovation is that people with similar needs in different parts of the country, or sometimes a local area, are experiencing very different forms of care, based on different assumptions, different sorts of providers and, crucially, different rights of access" (Walker, 1995, p 210).

The problems of coordination

The continuing division of responsibilities between the NHS and local authority social services departments for health and social care services for older people exacerbates problems of coordination, particularly when older people's needs cross the boundaries between different service domains. The local reviews of needs and provision for long-term NHS care are reported to have led to a hardening of attitudes towards professional and service responsibilities and less flexibility at the margins between NHS and local authority services (LGMB, 1997). Funding pressures have forced ever tighter boundaries to be drawn around service remits and responsibilities – what has been called the 'Red Sea Syndrome' (Berman et al, 1990), as the risk increases of older people falling into cracks between services.

It is not uncommon for older people with complex needs to receive services from a number of different sources (Audit Commission, 1997). This is a particular problem in relation to intimate personal care needs, where threats to privacy are likely to have a considerable impact on the acceptability of external services. It is also highly problematic in situations where service needs change rapidly as an older person's condition deteriorates or improves. For example, a recent study of services for older people suffering hip fractures concluded that "many patients ... have multiple problems and receive care from a number of different professionals in a number of different locations. And yet, all too often, no one is clearly placed to provide this co-ordination.... The result is care that is fragmented and disjointed, with adverse effects on the outcomes for patients" (Audit Commission, 1995, p 55).

A reduction in citizenship rights?

Despite the universality with which the NHS is popularly associated, there is no doubt that the professional judgements of doctors and nurses were traditionally major determinants of access to publicly funded long-term care services for older people. Between 1983 and 1993, the availability of social security payments to fund institutional care meant that transparent and legally enforceable civil rights replaced professional judgements, at least for the poorest older people; and also furnished the dominant basis for obtaining access to these particular long-term care services. With the 1993 'community care' changes, professional judgements once more gained prominence, but now accompanied by the formal managerial processes associated with assessment. The cumulative impact of these changes has been to shift a substantial element of responsibility for funding from public to private domains, with publicly funded long-term care services now available to only the very poorest older people.

Moreover, despite the rhetoric of 'consumerism' which has dominated public debate and policies over the past decade, there is little evidence that the choices available to older people who receive services through local authority social services departments have increased markedly. The development of a wide range of independent sector providers of residential and nursing home care during the 1980s was patchy, the development of a wide range of independent sector domiciliary service providers during the 1990s even more so. Social services care managers, purchasing services on behalf of their older clients, are restricted in their range of options by the market and organisational constraints described above. Meanwhile, growing income inequalities among older people since the late 1970s (Hancock and Weir, 1994) have also depressed the purchasing power of a substantial minority of older people who might otherwise have sought to meet their care needs through purchasing in the private market. The incomes of single, older and female pensioners, precisely those groups most at risk of needing health and social care services, have increased considerably more slowly than average (Falkingham, 1998). Even where older people are able to purchase domestic and other services in the private market, this often represents a considerable financial sacrifice. Moreover there is little evidence that the private purchase of services enables older people to exercise consumer power, to withdraw their custom in cases of poor service or otherwise alter supplier behaviour (Wilson, 1994).

The capacity to exercise choice of course depends upon older people's knowledge of the options which are potentially available to them, but it is far from clear that this kind of information is widely available and understood. Studies of older people on the margins of admission to residential care (Allen et al, 1992) and of people discharged from hospital after a stroke (Baldock and Ungerson, 1994) found that few were aware of the assessment and care management processes they had supposedly undergone, who their designated care manager was, how the services they received were organised, or how much they were likely to be charged for them.

Future prospects

A number of future developments promise to address some of the problems identified in this chapter. First, the Royal Commission on Long-Term Care for the Elderly is currently considering future funding arrangements, including the appropriate mix of public and private responsibilities for funding long-term care; hopefully the Commission's recommendations will provide the basis for wide-ranging public debate.

Second, proposed modifications to the NHS quasi-market also emphasise the importance of partnership at all levels with local authority social services departments. All NHS organisations will be placed under a new duty to work 'in partnership' with local authority services. Primary Care Groups, which will replace GP Fundholding and commission hospital and community health services for up to 100,000 patients, will be required to have social services representation on their governing bodies; health authorities will be required to include proposals for the joint development of services with the local authority in their strategic Health Improvement Programmes; and NHS regional offices will lead and monitor local action to strengthen partnerships across health and social care (DoH, 1997b). Proposals for Health Action Zones – wider interorganisational alliances to promote health gain – also place great emphasis on closer collaboration between NHS and local authority services (DoH, 1997b).

More generally, the government is giving considerable emphasis to the development of new strategies to deal with problems of poor coordination between services and the limited range of service options available to frail older people. Many of these are currently in the form of pilot projects and schemes, albeit in some instances covering very large geographical areas and population bases. Health Action Zones (DoH, 1997b) will pioneer new cross-sectoral alliances (including the NHS, local authorities, and the voluntary and private commercial sectors) with the aim of tackling local problems of deprivation and poor health. Within local government services,

'Best Value' pilot schemes will combine new approaches to setting and monitoring the standards of local services with active local participation and democratic accountability. Third, the 'Better Government for Older People' initiative is similarly piloting new service partnerships, again with a strong emphasis on user involvement and accountability.

However, it is important that the lessons from innovative schemes such as these are learnt, disseminated widely and absorbed into mainstream policy and practice. Failure to do so will simply increase the inequalities and variability in services available to older people in different localities. In particular, it will be vitally important to extend more widely experiences from pilot schemes of involving older people themselves in discussions and debates about the kinds of services they want; about the financial contributions they are able and willing to make, in the context of lifetime histories of contributing to the welfare state through their economic and care-giving activities; and about the ways in which services are delivered. There is now considerable experience of involving older people – even those who are isolated and housebound – in discussions about the planning and provision of services (Bewley and Glendinning, 1994; Thornton and Tozer, 1995; Barnes, 1997). Moreover, this experience extends beyond consumer-oriented consultation on a narrow range of issues, to the involvement of older people in the development, management and operation of services, as well as in the assessment of need. "The only way that frail and vulnerable service users can be assured of influence and power over service provision is if they ... are guaranteed a voice.... This would, in turn, ensure that services actually reflected their needs" (Walker, 1994, p 15).

THREE

The social insurance model of care for older people in Germany

Michaela Schunk

Introduction

This chapter describes the introduction and implementation of the new system of social insurance for people with long-term care needs in Germany. Long-term health and social care needs in old age were largely excluded from coverage by the German sickness insurance scheme from its inception in 1911 until the late 1980s, on the grounds that they are normal manifestations of the ageing body and do not require active medical treatment. This traditional separation of people with long-term care needs into the 'deserving' acutely ill and the 'undeserving' chronically ill and long-term frail came under increasing criticism, on a number of counts.

First, there has long been a lack of interest on the part of health professionals in treating the chronic illness and multi-morbidity experienced by old people. The marginalisation of geriatrics and psychogeriatrics, which are not regarded as medical specialties in German medical training, contributed significantly to the lack of provision and service development (Görres, 1992; 1996). Second, there was a serious lack of collective provision for the (rising) costs of long-term care; this led to older people having to 'spend down' their lifetime savings and subsequently experiencing discrimination and stigmatisation when they eventually had to claim social assistance (Dieck, 1990). Moreover, the costs and lost earnings experienced by informal carers were not considered a public responsibility.

Third, financial help with the costs of long-term care were fragmented between a number of different funders – some very limited entitlements under the sickness insurance scheme, the locally-operated means-tested social assistance schemes and older people themselves. These fragmented funding responsibilities resulted in equally fragmented long-term care services. Service development was very slow compared to other industrialised countries. Service providers offered only a limited range of services – nursing care which was related to or arose from medical treatment, personal care, and domestic home help. These services were tailored to the very limited categories of services which could be reimbursed under the sickness insurance scheme (Dieck and Garms-Homolová, 1991). Without any funding from insurance entitlements and with social assistance recipients as their only clients, the very few day care and respite care services delivered outside the private home – what is termed 'semi-institutional' care in Germany – were expensive and attracted only a few privately paying clients. In summary, the consequences of these very fragmented entitlements to the costs of long-term care were piecemeal care provision, a strong pull towards institutionalised care, catastrophic costs for older people needing long-term care and a lack of social security and social protection for informal carers.

On the provider side, the traditional service provider organisations were six leading welfare organisations. Serving particular groups of people according to their religious, social or political affiliations, these have long formed a 'virtual cartel' (Lorenz, 1994) in local welfare markets. As independent and non-profit organisations, they were traditionally given priority over public providers in delivering welfare services, but their policies often reflected their own organisational interests rather than the needs of clients. As a result, standard services were often duplicated and there was little incentive to diversify or introduce innovative new services (Geiser and Rosendahl, 1995).

In 1994 a new care insurance scheme was introduced to cover the risks of 'care dependency'. Care insurance joins the other four German social insurance schemes – unemployment, sickness, accident and retirement. The new insurance scheme provides a number of non-means-tested benefits for home care, day care, respite care and institutional care. Although the care insurance scheme does not include a cash benefit paid directly to informal carers, a new home care cash benefit is explicitly meant to be handed over to the carer. It is tax-free for both the older person and the carer. The insurance scheme also provides benefits to cover an annual period of respite care and pays the pension and accident insurance contributions of an informal carer.

Under the new care insurance scheme, guidelines have been drawn up to create a single, clear definition of 'care dependency' and establish different degrees of its severity. These guidelines are now applied across both the care insurance and social assistance schemes and their various programmes. Policy debates on the concept of 'care dependency' and clarification of statutory and professional responsibilities in the wake of the care insurance reforms have also drawn attention to the relative underdevelopment of geriatric and psychogeriatric medical and nursing care and geriatric rehabilitation in Germany; it is slowly being acknowledged that long-term frailty in old age is not a static condition but can be ameliorated. Indeed, assessments for care insurance explicitly include consideration of the feasibility of (psycho)geriatric rehabilitation and what has become known as 'activating care', in order to maintain or improve health status or slow down further deterioration.

The care insurance scheme must be seen in the context of pressing cost constraints and incentives to shift (albeit limited) costs from the sickness insurance and social assistance schemes. The objective of introducing a clear, uniform entitlement to care services and/or partial payment for care-related costs needs to be evaluated against the early evidence of the programme's implementation. What impact has care insurance had so far on care provision for older people in Germany? Despite its significance in conferring social insurance entitlements to people with care needs, considerable shortcomings can be identified. These shortcomings centre on the overall adequacy of benefits, limitations on the choices available to older people and their families, inequities and inconsistencies in the assessment process and continuing gaps in the range, coordination, and quality of services.

Introducing care insurance

During the 1970s there were a number of attempts to develop coherent policies to deal with the increasing volume of long-term care needed by frail older people. These efforts were prompted by growing awareness of demographic changes and the associated demands for services and by the pressures of fiscal retrenchment. The latter pressures in particular led to a need to control rising demand and associated costs in the health sector and to curb the pressures of long-term care costs on the social assistance schemes.

The process of policy formation took some time (see Alber, 1996, for a detailed account). Care insurance was eventually introduced in 1994 as the fifth social insurance scheme in the German welfare state. It established a single definition of 'care dependency' and provides cover against the contingency risk of 'care dependency' for all citizens. Germany has therefore once again adopted a 'third way' (Schmidt, 1988, p 97) of providing social security. Unlike the Nordic countries, where long-term care is tax-financed and for the most part provided by the public sector, and unlike countries like the US and the UK where long-term care is privately funded or relies on means-tested programmes, "the social insurance model may be considered a compromise between a transfer model and a market model" (Alber, 1996).

The care insurance scheme is financed by adding a further 1.7% of gross earnings to the social insurance contributions which are traditionally spilt in half between employers and employees. However, because of the staunch resistance of employers' interest groups to any additional wage costs, the employers' costs have been compensated by the loss of one day's statutory paid holiday, thereby effectively shifting the burden of financing entirely on to employees. Thus in 1994, the social insurance contributions of employees (pensions, accident, unemployment, health and care) constituted about 20% of gross earnings (Clasen, 1994). Retirement pensioners receive half their contributions from their pension insurance schemes and unemployed people receive their full contribution rate from unemployment insurance.

Participation in the care insurance scheme is mandatory for everyone who has sickness insurance coverage, whether statutory or private. All private care insurance schemes are legally required to offer coverage, contributions and benefits on terms which are equivalent to the statutory scheme. Membership of both sickness and care insurance are near-universal, with people being insured in either the statutory or an equivalent private insurance scheme. From 1 January 1997, people claiming social assistance have also been covered by the statutory care insurance scheme; prior to this, people who were not insured and who had no private means were entitled to benefits equivalent to those provided by care insurance, but financed by the social assistance board.

Care insurance: regulations, entitlements and benefits

The care insurance scheme provides cash benefits, benefits in kind for home care services, day care and respite care and the costs of residential or nursing home care. The scheme was phased in between 1 January 1994 and 1 July 1996. In the first stage, contributions of 1% had to be paid from 1 January 1994 and benefits, which were limited to home care services, started on 1 April 1994. From 1 July 1996, contribution levels were raised to 1.7% of gross income and benefits were extended to cover the costs of institutional care (see Klie, 1995, for detailed documentation of the care insurance legislation).

Contracts and price regulation

Provider organisations must register with the care insurance funds, thereby entering into a contractual agreement covering the professional conduct of their business. Subsequently, reimbursement contracts between the care insurance funds and provider organisations may be agreed; these set out the terms and prices under which the services offered by the provider organisations are eligible for reimbursement under the care insurance scheme.

The procedures for entering into provision contracts are relatively open and allow, for example, private individuals to register as service providers. In a significant new development, the care insurance legislation now gives priority over public sector providers not only to the six leading welfare organisations (as under the former arrangements) but also to non-profit and commercial providers. This new competitive scenario may eventually stimulate major changes among service provider organisations and, in particular, challenge the 'cosy collaboration' between the leading traditional welfare service provider organisations and public authorities at local levels. However, as will be discussed below, it may be much more difficult to bring about coordination and cooperation between the private, voluntary and public provider organisations to ensure a user-friendly, responsive mix of local services.

For the reimbursement contracts between providers and the care insurance funds, all service elements have to be specified and priced and care insurance funds are required to make this information available to the consumer. For services such as institutional care, respite care and day care, a clear line is drawn between 'care-related' costs and the so-called 'board and lodging' costs which are not covered by care insurance. Unlike the former system of funding, once prices are set they are binding for the contract period and cannot be increased to cover any increases in real costs. This is intended to keep down the prices of services and introduce competition into the service market.

Prices must not include investment and building costs. Under the care insurance legislation, public funding of these costs has become the responsibility of the regional governments (*Länder*). The Länder have therefore potentially gained considerable influence, as gatekeepers of capital service developments. However, the allocation of finance to promote comprehensive, accessible and high quality service networks is entirely at their discretion; this may eventually lead to greater territorial inequity in the service infrastructure.

'Care dependency guidelines' and the assessment procedure

Under previous arrangements, the recommendation of the local medical practitioner was crucial in determining whether the social assistance board would agree to meet the costs of institutional care. Now claimants for care insurance benefits are assessed by a 'medical board', an officially independent consultancy service financed jointly by the sickness and care insurance funds. Entitlement to care insurance benefits depends on the assessment of the medical board and the discretionary decision of the care insurance fund itself. This decision can be challenged, formally reviewed and eventually brought to the social court.

The care insurance legislation included a requirement that a commission, representing all the major health and welfare organisations at federal level, should be established to draw up so-called "care dependency guidelines" (*Pflegebedürftigkeits-Richtlinien*). These guidelines, which are standardised across the country, establish clear criteria for assessing 'care dependency' and its degree of severity. The severity of the 'care dependency' in turn determines the level of benefits paid.

The grade of 'care dependency' is determined by the length of time for which assistance with a range of basic activities is required each day. The activities covered by the 'care dependency' assessment are personal care, eating and mobility; any help needed with domestic or household tasks is given lower priority. In June 1997 the care dependency guidelines were revised and now include a guide to the length of time for which help is likely to be required for each type of activity. These so-called 'time corridors', with upper and lower limits of the length of time likely to be taken in helping with each task, are designed to aid assessors' estimates of the amount of time for which care is required and improve the consistency of assessments (KDA, 1997).

Care insurance funds are also legally required to assess claimants' needs for rehabilitation services and to forward any such requirements to the sickness insurance funds which are responsible for payment. The care insurance assessment can therefore result in recommendations for rehabilitation services (financed by the sickness insurance); this is particularly likely when the claimant is assessed as not sufficiently 'care dependent' to meet the minimum care insurance scheme threshold.

Benefits

Where the assessment confirms eligibility for care insurance benefits, the claimant can choose between a cash payment or benefits in kind – home care or day care services up to a specified value. It is also possible to choose a combination of both cash and service benefits. The choice of the cash option depends on whether appropriate home care can be arranged privately.

The monthly benefits are graded according to the degree of 'care dependency' (Table 3.1):

Table 3.1: Main benefits of care insurance schemes

For personal care and home help services in the household:
- if arranged privately (cash option):

grade 1:	400 DM	(£133)
grade 2:	800 DM	(£266)
grade 3:	1,300 DM	(£433)

- if provided by approved provider service organisation (benefit in kind option):

grade 1:	750 DM	(£250)
grade 2:	1,800 DM	(£600)
grade 3:	2,800 DM	(£933)

- or any combination of the two, with the chosen 'mix' binding for 6 months

Use of day care or night care facilities, including transportation costs **(counts as a proportion of the 'benefit in kind' option):**

grade 1:	750 DM	(£250)
grade 2:	1,500 DM	(£500)
grade 3:	2,100 DM	(£700)

Respite care **(annual benefit, informal carer must have been main carer for at least the previous 12 months):**

- for use of approved provider service (benefit in kind):

all grades up to:	2,800 DM	(£933)

- or private arrangement with substitute carer (cash benefit):

grade 1:	400 DM	(£133)
grade 2:	800 DM	(£266)
grade 3:	1,300 DM	(£433)

Contribution to the costs of equipment/house adaptations:
• or reimbursement of lost earnings and/or travel expenses of substitute carers:
• for equipment (if the equipment required is not available for rent from care insurance funds):

60 DM (£20)

• for housing adaptations (depending on means test):

5,000 DM (£1666)

Pension and accident insurance contributions for informal carers

The care insurance pays the retirement pension and accident insurance contributions of the family carers of older people who qualify for care insurance. Informal carers must be providing care for at least 14 hours a week and receive no other payment for their care services, apart from the care insurance 'cash' benefit. The amount of the pension contributions is calculated using a projected wage (minimum 1,138 DM [£379] to maximum 3,416 DM [£1,138] for West Germany), depending on the grade of care dependency and the amount of care provided. The care insurance also offers free training courses for informal carers.

Institutional care

The care insurance covers some of the costs of institutional care, up to a maximum of 2,800 DM a month. Elderly people living in private households who are assessed as less 'care dependent' than grade 3 are not thought to require institutional care. However, if they do choose to enter institutional care, they may contribute any grade 1 or 2 benefit they receive towards the costs of institutional care. For current residents (many of whom entered institutions before the care insurance was introduced), institutions receive a monthly benefit, graded according to the degree of 'care dependency': grade 1: 2,000 DM (£666); grade 2: 2,500 DM (£833); grade 3: 2,800 DM (£933); exceptional needs: 33,00 DM (£1,100). Social Assistance Boards are obliged to continue payment for current residents in institutional care who not assessed as eligible for care insurance benefits (PIB, 1996).

Take-up of care insurance benefits: claims, outcomes and coverage

After four years of operation, the care insurance scheme has been judged to be successful overall. Take-up rates are consistent with earlier estimates of the prevalence of 'care dependency' in Germany (Schneekloth, 1996). The overall level of expenditure on benefits associated with 'care dependency' has increased substantially (BAS, 1998). For example, the total value of benefits to support home care arrangements has increased ten-fold, compared to the spending on means-tested social assistance benefits before the introduction of care insurance. At the same time, the number of people claiming social assistance because of their care needs has decreased.

By mid-1997, about 1.7 million people received care insurance benefits (BAS, 1998). This figure includes about 90,000 beneficiaries who have taken up mandatory care insurance with private insurers. Care insurance beneficiaries living in private households outnumber those living in institutions by three to one. Of the beneficiaries in private households, 46% have been assessed at 'care dependency' grade 1, 42% at grade 2 and 12% at the highest, grade 3. About one third, 29%, of all applications to statutory care insurance funds were unsuccessful. This proportion of unsuccessful applications is considerably higher than to the private care insurance funds, where only 16% of applicants were denied benefits.

The care insurance scheme gives successful claimants in private households the choice between a benefit in cash to support informal care arrangements and a benefit in kind for care services provided by professional formal provider organisations. Although the value of the 'cash option' is only about half that of the benefit in kind, an overwhelming majority of successful applicants choose the cash benefit. In 1995, about 80% of claimants in private households chose the 'cash' option, 10% the benefit in kind, and 10% a combination of the two (PIB, 1995). The number of people choosing a combination of 'cash' and 'kind' is rising, according to a recent review of the care insurance scheme (BAS, 1998, p 22).

The care insurance benefits also include the payment of pension contributions for informal carers. In 1997, about 500,000 informal carers received such contributions, the majority (90%) of them women (BAS, 1998). Two aims of the care insurance scheme, the promotion of care at home and improved social security benefits for informal carers, therefore appear to have been achieved. However, in what has effectively been a curtailing of benefits, the annual respite care benefit now only consists of a payment equivalent to the cash benefit rates, unless higher wage losses and/or travel expenses can be claimed by the substitute informal carer or professional services are being used.

The impact of care insurance on the care of older people in Germany: "A field of experimentation in cost control" (Dieck, 1994, p 265)

The German care insurance scheme aims both to alleviate, at least in part, the risks of financial hardship arising from care dependency and to redistribute significantly the costs of long-term care from the tax-financed social assistance scheme to a contribution-financed insurance model (Alber, 1996; Landenberger, 1995). However, there is considerable concern about the long-term financial viability of the care insurance scheme in the context of continued demographic ageing and labour market pressures.

> **The dynamics of social security systems once they have been established ... [create] ... the difficulty of cost control and control of service expansion. Efforts to control the rise of costs of health insurance in recent years have not been very effective.... Cost control within such systems of social security may well become more and more difficult... (Dieck, 1990, pp 110-11)**

The care insurance scheme contains four distinctive mechanisms to control rising costs. First, care insurance benefits have fixed ceilings and are not open-ended entitlements dependent on needs. Unlike the other German social insurance schemes, which can raise their contribution rates according to increases in expenditure, the care insurance contribution rate of 1.7% can be changed by only Federal legislation. This is a departure from the principle of full coverage of all needs and costs which are seen in the health insurance and accident insurance schemes (Landenberger, 1995).

Second, the 'care dependency' guidelines which govern assessment and entitlement to care insurance benefits are formulated by a consortium of purchasers' representatives (the care insurance funds, sickness insurance funds and social assistance boards), provider organisations, professional bodies, and user organisations. While the purchasers share relatively common interests, there is more diversity among the other groups and this has the effect of shifting the bargaining power within the consortium to the care insurance funds. Moreover, the Federal Ministry must approve the 'care dependency' entitlement guidelines and has thus retained not only processual but also substantive regulatory powers. The care insurance legislation does not include a time limit on these exceptional Federal government powers, which do not exist for any other branch of social insurance in Germany (Igl, 1996).

Third, the assessing body, the medical board, is jointly financed by the sickness insurance and the care insurance funds. Staffed by doctors and nurses, and situated at arm's length from the administration of the care insurance funds, the medical board acts as a gatekeeper for care insurance entitlements. However, it is the care insurance scheme which actually makes decisions about eligibility, on the basis of recommendations from the medical board. Despite the elaborate and closely specified assessment guidelines, assessing the degree of 'care dependency' necessarily includes subjective elements and this allows assessors to tighten or lower their threshold criteria according to the financial agendas set by the care insurance funds. In fact significant variations have been found between the various care insurance funds in the percentage of unsuccessful applications and in the assignment of the different grades of care dependency (Jonas, 1996).

Finally, the cash benefit option, albeit paid at a much lower rate than the value of benefits in kind, provides a major incentive for home-based, family care; this will reduce overall levels of care costs. A further consequence of the cash benefit option is likely to be a reduction in the participation of (predominately) women in the formal labour market (Landenberger, 1995).

A number of other consequences of the German care insurance model can be anticipated. Although 'care dependency' is now officially acknowledged and consistently defined, it also risks being in some ways marginalised from the other German social welfare and social protection systems. Previously a number of the social security schemes included some fragmented provision for 'care dependency' at their margins; it is likely that they will now abandon their former financial responsibilities. For the person with care needs, the only option will now be to apply for care insurance benefits, with their relatively high qualifying threshold; a complex process of application, assessment, non-eligibility and reassessments may be triggered.

Because of the duty of the assessing medical board to consider rehabilitation needs as part of the assessment of care dependency and make recommendations about treatment to the sickness insurance funds, there is now greater emphasis on the rehabilitation of older people within the sickness insurance system than before. Nevertheless, both individual entitlements to rehabilitation treatment and the funding of such services are precarious and depend upon the overall financial commitments of the sickness insurance funds. Since health research in Germany is still poorly developed, it is difficult to evaluate possible changes in the provision of rehabilitative services since the introduction of the care insurance (Landenberger, 1995).

The care insurance scheme contains no incentives for health and care professionals to collaborate or plan services together. The only care planning is contained in the assessment by the medical board, and this is geared towards determining benefit eligibility rather than obtaining a comprehensive overview of an individual's needs and how they might best be met. The available service options remain, as before, characterised by a narrow range of standardised services. Only the discretionary activities of some quality-oriented professionals may offer an holistic and individual approach to individual needs assessment and care planning.

Price regulation and the quality of services

In relation to the care insurance service benefits 'in kind', there is no clear specification of those elements of care needs which are supposed to be covered. The legislation allows service providers, particularly those offering day and institutional care services, to offer 'additional care services' and charge extra fees for these. There is concern that this will encourage provider organisations to remove some elements of social care from the basic service 'package' and instead provide these as 'additional' services for which they can then make additional charges. Some social aspects of care – providing social support and recreational activities, for example – thus risk becoming a privilege for more affluent older people who can afford the additional charges. However, the first amendment to the care insurance legislation stipulated that social activities and social care elements of institutional care are included in the coverage of care as long as their costs do not exceed the benefit maximum insurance reimbursement (PIB, 1996). Yet there is increasing evidence of serious difficulties being experienced by the providers of institutional care in maintaining high quality services under the tight budget imposed by the capped care insurance benefits (KDA, 1998).

The reimbursement agreements between care insurance funds and provider organisations also set the prices of board and lodgings in institutional settings, although these are not included in the care insurance reimbursements and frail older people must meet these from their own private means. Although this represents an attempt to regulate the costs which older people themselves have to meet on entering institutional care, it is mainly intended to control the expenditure which falls on the social assistance boards, which still have to pay these board and lodgings costs for the poorest older people.

The care insurance benefits are flat rate and not indexed to inflation, so their value is likely to decrease over time. There is therefore a risk that the rising costs of care, particularly in institutional settings, will soon exceed the value of the care insurance benefit. However, current debates are mainly concerned with the effects of increased price regulation on the quality of care. Charges for institutional care must now be set prospectively, purchasers (the care insurance funds) have gained considerable power over the setting and regulation of prices, and prices may not include elements of capital costs. In contrast, the regulation of standards of quality is weak. There are no legally defined guidelines on staffing levels in institutional care homes at national level, and wide variations exist in the standards which are set as part of the price negotiations at Länder level (Allemeyer, 1994a). It is indeed very likely that the strong cost containment measures built into the care insurance scheme will inhibit attempts to improve standards and quality of care. Although quality guidelines have been formulated at a national level (Klie, 1995), these so far cover only home care services and mainly specify the qualifications required of staff; in any case, these were already in operation in the provider contracts used by the sickness insurance funds in relation to the few care services funded by the sickness insurance scheme.

Who benefits most?

A comparison of the incomes of social assistance recipients with the costs of institutional care showed that, even with the care insurance benefit, about 45% of former claimants will continue to claim social assistance benefits, albeit at a much lower rate (Peukert, 1993, in Alber, 1996). Allemeyer (1994b) calculates that in Hamburg a much higher proportion (60 to 80%) of the residents of institutional care who were claiming social assistance will continue to do so. However, his analysis shows that these will mainly be residents with the highest levels of 'care dependency' (grade 3), for whom care costs are highest. Thus 'care dependency' is likely to continue to create a risk of poverty for a substantial group of older people, with the associated stigmatisation and marginalisation of having to 'spend down' assets and claim social assistance.

Allemeyer also estimated that between 60 and 80% of social assistance recipients who had been receiving home care services would probably have to continue claiming the costs of this care from the social assistance scheme (Allemeyer, 1994a), because many of them would not qualify for care insurance benefits on the grounds that they mainly needed help with domestic and household tasks rather than personal care. On the other hand, the care needs of those who do qualify for care insurance benefits are much higher than is covered by even the (higher level) insurance benefit in kind. When compared with the current prices of standard service assignments, only half the amount of care needed to qualify for benefits according to the care dependency guidelines is covered by the benefit in kind, at each of the three grades.

Alber (1996) argues that the care insurance scheme favours the middle classes who were hitherto above the income limit for the social assistance scheme, while lower income groups continue to have access to the social assistance scheme. Thus the overall distributional effects of the care insurance, which is funded by contributions from all income groups, effectively favours the affluent (Dudey, 1991). However, there are arguments against this conclusion. Alber (1996) argues that the care insurance scheme is more progressive in its redistributive effects; higher income classes contribute proportionately more to the scheme but receive only the same, flat-rate benefits. Winters (1991) has argued that the stigmatising effects of having to claim social assistance (which includes the assessment of adult children's incomes) has been replaced by a qualitatively different entitlement to an insurance benefit. This, he argues, particularly favours the lower to middle income groups just above the social assistance threshold, who were most at risk of becoming impoverished as a consequence of their needs for care. Moreover, Winters points to the redistributional effects between people who become care dependent in old age and those who do not and, because of women's greater longevity, between men and women.

Will gaps in the service mix remain unchanged?

With the aim of containing costs, increasing importance is given to the provision of closely specified services, defined and tailored to the conditions under which they are reimbursed by the care insurance funds. As a result, services continue to be highly segmented, tightly prescribed and inflexible (Dieck and Garms-Homolová, 1991). The range of care services which will be reimbursed by the care insurance scheme is therefore not likely to develop a diverse and varied mix. Although there is increasing choice for older people over which particular provider organisations they receive services from, they still have little choice in the types of services which are on offer (Evers, 1995). Moreover, there are still very few information, advice or brokerage services to help people without informal carers or friends who can help to arrange care services and optimise the limited choices available. Very frail, isolated, and disoriented older people are at a particular disadvantage here. Moreover, because the threshold for qualifying for care insurance benefits is high, those in the early stages of 'care dependency', who might benefit from preventive services, are likely to be excluded altogether; again there will be no incentive for service providers to develop these services because they will not be reimbursed.

Advice and information services and other so called 'soft services' (visiting, social or recreational services) are not included in the services covered by the care insurance. Their availability remains largely at the discretion of municipalities and Länder and dependent on their particular political priorities and financial commitments. The development of 'soft' services in response to particular local needs will therefore inevitably lead to territorial inequalities. It has already been pointed out that the introduction of care insurance has led to a decrease in the influence which local municipalities could exercise over service planning, because their role as major funders of services (through the local social assistance schemes) has diminished. Municipalities have also not obtained any increase in their power to influence the range or coordination of services available locally (Evers, 1996). In contrast, the leverage of the Länder over service development has been enhanced with the introduction of care insurance. However, their new responsibilities for meeting the capital elements of services may not lead to greater flexibility and responsiveness. Allemayer (1994a) argues that responsive service development is more likely to happen in a system where capital costs are integrated into service prices, instead of being diverted to a separate funding body. Moreover the former activities of the Länder in planning services have been criticised for being too rigid and insufficiently responsive to local variations (Stratman and Korte, 1993).

The easy option: the cash benefit

The care insurance cash benefit has also been criticised. It is only half the value of the benefit in kind that is paid if professional care services carry out the care. Under the care insurance legislation, the insurance funds are allowed to grant the cash benefit only if the necessary care can be secured. This forms part of the assessment carried out by the medical board. In addition, everyone who opts for the cash benefit only is required to undergo regular visits by a professional service provider of their choice to check on the quality of the care they are receiving.

These measures have been criticised as being too weak to guarantee good quality care by informal carers. It has been argued that receipt of the cash benefit should have been made dependent on the willingness of the informal carer to participate in more active forms of quality assurance (Naegele and Igl, 1993; Evers, 1995). The cash benefit has also been criticised as being too low to allow informal carers to purchase additional care services on an ad hoc basis, to relieve them of some of the work of care-giving (Evers, 1995).

On the one hand, the conditions attached to receipt of the cash benefit allow the needs of family care-givers to be contained and remain invisible. On the other hand, potential risks and problems associated with intensive informal care-giving are unlikely to be prevented. Power inequalities and conflicts of interest between an older person and younger family care-givers may lead to situations in which one or other opts for the cash benefit, regardless of the fact that the other might benefit from a certain amount of service inputs in kind.

The choice of the cash benefit by 80% of care insurance beneficiaries reflects – and further reinforces – the limited options and acceptability of formal service provision. The large, established service provider organisations in particular fail to attract clients because they are too traditional and unresponsive to changes in the characteristics of frail older people and their needs (Hegner, 1991). The low take-up of the formal service option may also be explained by the legacy of 'cultural maps' in care consumption (Evers, 1996), particularly the traditional lack of entitlements to services and the consequently low levels of home care and day care service provision. It may take some time for older people and their families to develop trust in formal services and experience their benefits, rather than viewing them as a potential intrusion into familiar patterns of family care-giving.

As long as the cash option in its current form continues to be popular, there will be little pressure for additional public expenditure to develop a network of supplementary services.

Much ado about nothing? The care insurance reforms revisited

The care insurance reforms introduced a substantial number of non-means-tested benefits for people needing care and significant new options for people to choose and design their own care arrangements. As a social risk covered by social insurance entitlements, 'care dependency' has thus moved across the insurance/assistance divide which characterises the German social security system, to become a national programme with standardised assessment procedures. However, within the scheme a number of weaknesses have been identified. These are the inadequacy of the value of insurance benefits, both cash and in kind; the risk of inequities in care provision arising from the introduction of charges for additional care services; and the potential decrease in the actual value of benefits as they remain constant while inflation and costs rise. Furthermore, there is growing evidence of and concern about the variable interpretation of the care dependency guidelines in different regions and between different care insurance funds.

A number of problems in coordinating services have been identified. First, responsibilities for service planning are only poorly covered by the care insurance legislation, although some innovative attempts to improve planning at local and regional levels have been reported (Geiser and Rosendahl, 1995). Second, continuing boundary disputes between the sickness and care insurance funds about responsibilities for rehabilitation services continue to leave a substantial number of people without entitlements to such services. Third, the legislation gives no incentives to care insurance funds to act as anything but purchasers. There are few incentives to promote collaboration between provider organisations or to encourage the participation of users in service evaluation and monitoring the quality of care. Fourth, the emphasis on individual social rights in the care insurance scheme inhibits attempts to introduce case management and coordination of services for individual users, other than through the standardised assessment for benefit eligibility.

The substantial difference between the value of the cash benefit and the benefit in kind reinforces the boundaries between professional and non-professional care. The care insurance scheme encourages the provision of care by informal carers. Indeed, the most substantial extension of benefits through the care insurance is the cash benefit for informal home care arrangements. However, informal carers remain hidden in the private realm. Little is known about the processes of decision making regarding care arrangements, what factors influence the choice of cash or kind types of benefits, and how the benefit options affect relationships between the older person and the care-giver or the quality of care provided. The fact that entitlement rests with the older person and the benefits are assigned to them leaves informal carers in the shadow, without any direct entitlement to the cash benefit and only 'secondary' entitlements to social security protection of their own. The fact that 80% of insurance beneficiaries choose the cash benefit strikingly reflects the continuing profound alienation of so many older people from professional services. It is still unclear to what extent these attitudes are the result of the continuing unresponsiveness of services or of cultural and historical factors.

The introduction of the care insurance scheme in Germany represents some limited extension to the social rights of older people with substantial care needs and to the social protection of people (mainly women) who are engaged in informal caring activities. However, a much more comprehensive approach to care reform would be required in order to remedy the inadequate range of formal service provision, the gulf between care provided within the family and care provided by external professional providers and the poor coordination of services at both micro- and macro-levels. Yet because of the political and institutional structures of the German social security system, a broader and more radical approach has been impeded. Overall, care insurance represents a complicated compromise to contain the costs of care dependency. The prospects for more substantial changes are not promising, partly because of the constraints of the policy making process and partly because of the German economic crisis and the growing political pressures to curb, inter alia, care insurance contribution rates.

Note

Benefit rates are those current in 1997 (BAS, 1998). Rates are converted from DM into £ by factor 3.

FOUR

Long-term care in The Netherlands: public funding and private provision within a universalistic welfare state

Jan Coolen and Sylvia Weekers

Introduction

Chronically ill and disabled older people often need comprehensive packages of services, either simultaneously or consecutively. However, comparative studies have argued that the production and delivery of effective support for elderly people is hindered by administrative, organisational and financial segmentation in health and social care systems (Jamieson, 1993). Such segmentation creates obstacles in providing 'coherent support' or 'continuity of care' to very dependent older people (Jamieson, 1993), by restricting the coherence of government planning of services, coordination between service providers and freedom of choice for 'consumers' in a social care market.

This chapter explores changes in the structure of long-term care services in The Netherlands from the following viewpoints. First, it will describe how responsibilities for long-term care are fragmented across a number of boundaries: between national and local government, care and cash benefits, and between institutional and community based services. Second, the chapter will describe a number of policy strategies aimed at overcoming dysfunctional boundaries: the introduction of greater flexibility in service delivery (the ideology of 'tailor-made' solutions); the introduction of greater consumer choice through an experimental 'personal budget' scheme; and the provision of more support for independent living, through increased coherence in the provision of housing, care, technical aids and social assistance.

Finally, the chapter will review the consequences of these various strategies on the accessibility, quality and efficiency of care; and will discuss possible future developments in the balance of public and private responsibilities for long-term care.

The structure of health and social care services in The Netherlands

Basic pattern

The national government regulates the supply of health and social services, whose provision is delegated to independent (non-statutory), non-profit organisations (see Table 4.1). These organisations function within a framework of fixed budgets and quality standards set by the government and the regional health insurance companies. It is predominantly the managers and professionals of the non-profit provider organisations who control the micro-allocation of services to individual older people. However, recently a new system of needs-testing has been introduced, in which the functions of assessment and the matching of demand and supply are carried out by independent local or regional agencies, which are controlled by local governments and the health insurance companies.

Some competition between service providers has emerged as a result of attempts to introduce cost-effectiveness approaches in healthcare policy, but 'quasi-market' arrangements have developed slowly. Up until now, providers have not been subjected to a system of managed care that forces them to compete in terms of the quality and price ratios of services. Recently, the government has introduced elements of market competition into home care services, by allowing regional health authorities to contract with for-profit providers as well as with the established non-profit providers. However, this trend has slowed down following critical reviews from the national parliament, which found too many changes in home care provision, insufficient coordination and inadequate implementation.

A minority of older service users have been allowed to make use of 'cash benefits' in the form of a 'personal budget' with which to purchase their own services. This constitutes between only 3% and 5% of the total costs of long-term care for older people; most older people in need of care continue to receive services 'in kind'.

Within the realm of long-term care, the established distinction between health and social welfare services has become blurred. Home nursing and home help services, nursing homes and residential care homes are treated equally within a single regulatory and financial framework. The basic elements of long-term care services are:

- institutional care (nursing home and residential home), funded through a combination of the national care fund and user charges;
- community-based services (home nursing and home help) and intermediate care services, funded from the same sources as institutional care;
- adapted and sheltered housing, regulated by local government and provided by social housing organisations and residential homes;
- technical aids such as wheelchairs, which are provided by the local government;
- social welfare services, subsidised by local government.

Funding

Healthcare in The Netherlands is financed mainly through health insurance and taxation. A sharp distinction is made between 'cure'- and 'care'-related services. The costs of 'cure'-related services – primary healthcare and hospitals – are covered through three arrangements: social health insurance for people below a certain income level, which covers 63% of the population; health insurance for various categories of civil servants (5% coverage); and private health insurance schemes for the remaining 32% of the population with relatively high incomes. Membership of the social health insurance scheme is mandatory for all employees below a specific income level, claimants of social security (long-term unemployment, disability and social assistance) benefits, and old age pensioners who were admitted to social health insurance prior to age 65. It is based on contributions from employers and employees, supplemented by deficit funding from national government. Control of the fund rests with regional health insurance agencies, supervised by a national board.

The costs of long-term care are paid from a specific national care fund, based on the 1968 General Act on Exceptional Medical Expenses (AWBZ), which covers all citizens. Within fixed spending limits, this fund covers the planned supply and the needs-tested use of services for chronically ill, physically disabled and elderly people, people with severe learning disabilities and people with long-term psychiatric disorders. The national care fund is based on tax-related premiums from all citizens, supplemented by central government funding. The total budget is determined annually by the national government and subsequently divided between health planning regions.

In the total Dutch population of 15 million people, total healthcare ('cure' and 'care') expenditure adds up to approximately 10% of gross national product. Approximately one third of this expenditure is on services for people aged 65-plus, who constitute 13% of the population.

The use of formal services in The Netherlands is relatively high, resembling the situation in Scandinavian welfare states. As would be expected, formal service use is strongly related to the incidence of chronic health problems and disabilities, low income levels and low levels of informal support. In total, 61% of older people with moderate to very high levels of disability, concentrated in the 75-plus age group, benefit from publicly funded services (see Table 4.2). Low levels of informal support further influence the levels and type of services used (more institutional care as opposed to community-based services).

These patterns of service utilisation reflect a tendency towards a "hierarchical–compensatory model" (Cantor, 1980), where long-term care service use depends on interactions between 'need variables' and sociocultural variables such as household composition and, to a lesser extent, income.

Table 4.1: Planning and funding of long-term care in The Netherlands

Government level	Long-term care authorities	
Central government		• General budgetary framework for the provision of long-term care (non-profit services for elderly, disabled, chronically ill people) • Criteria for micro-allocation of services (needs assessment, selective targeting) • Quality standards for delivery and implementation of services
	National board for long-term care (*Ziekenfondsraad*)	• Control of national healthcare fund • Allocation of budgets to service providers based on national guidelines for the supply of services (eg, the number of nursing home beds and their regional distribution) and service prices (eg, acceptable costs of 7 x 24 hours care in a nursing home, per person per year)
Regional (provincial) government		• Overview of trends for need for long-term care • Demand for services, demand-supply relations • Advice on the structure of long-term care (supply, quality, innovation)
	Regional authority for long-term care (*Zorgkantoor*)	• Contracting with certified, non-profit providers as an intermediary agency between the national board and local or regional providers
Local government		• Overview of coordination between long-term care, adapted housing, transport facilities for disabled people, subsidised use of technical aids • Provision of technical aids for disability and mobility problems (wheelchairs, etc) • Regulation of adapted and sheltered housing and subsidies for social welfare services (meals on wheels etc) • Organisation of independent needs-assessment for long-term care, special housing and subsidised provision of technical aids (in cooperation with the regional authorities for long-term care)

Table 4.2: Use of long-term care in relation to level of disability (people above 75 years of age)

Degree of disability	None/ low (%)	Moderate (%)	High (%)	Very high (%)
Home help or home nursing	10	27	24	11
Home help and home nursing	0	1	10	8
Home for elderly people	6	16	35	51
Nursing home	0	0	7	18
Total	**16**	**44**	**76**	**88**

Notes

[1] Data from random surveys of the population aged over 75: n=1,226 (77% response rate).

[2] Moderate disability = inability to perform housekeeping tasks. (Very) high disability = inability to perform activities of daily living/ *and* inability to perform housekeeping tasks.

Stability and diversity

Overall, The Netherlands is characterised by relative stability in the funding and production of long-term care services, but diversity in the types and range of services which are supplied. Four policy factors contribute to this paradox. First, the distinction between 'cure' and 'care' is widespread. Hospitals have reduced the average length of stay, reflecting their core function within the domain of cure. Estimates of bed blocking in general hospitals are low, at less than 5% of total hospital-use days. Most healthcare regions have successfully created systems to transfer patients from 'cure' to 'care' services, in order to avoid hospital bed blocking and provide continuity across the boundaries between hospital and home. These include small-scale 'transmural' (intermediate) care projects, where qualified hospital nurses and primary healthcare professionals work together with chronically ill and very disabled older people.

Second, in all health regions there is increasing diversity in the range of long-term care services. New services have developed, such as short stay institutions, day care facilities and intensive home care. These are mainly targeted at older people who would otherwise require institutional care because of serious health problems, disabilities and low levels of informal support. However, in fact it is not this at-risk population which actually tends to receive these new services but other, less vulnerable older people, as the result of a process of 'demand creation'.

Third, sheltered housing has developed in a variety of ways, sometimes combined with social housing and at other times linked to institutional care. In addition, there has been a continued drive to create adapted housing for people with mobility or other disability problems, because it was assumed that this would enable older people to maintain an independent lifestyle. However, research has so far failed to demonstrate that either adapted or sheltered housing reduces the demand for institutional care or contains long-term care costs (Sociaal en Cultureel Planbureau, 1997). Some exceptions are found in programmes of 'very sheltered housing', which offer additional services and support above the regular community help.

Fourth, because of the important role of family and friends in providing long-term care, the government has introduced care allowance schemes which allow a closer integration of formal and informal care. Small-scale experiments have shown some interesting results: reduced rates of admission to institutional care; a more economic use of resources; and improved social integration of older people (Koedoot et al, 1991). Nevertheless, it is likely that family members' decisions to help elderly people are only marginally influenced by consideration of the financial incentives they might receive.

A universalistic welfare state

Despite the current debates on the planning and funding of long-term care, provision for both frail older and younger disabled people is still firmly rooted in a universalistic welfare state tradition. Four aspects of the Dutch system illustrate this tradition. First, central government regulates the supply of long-term care services through setting fixed (capped) budgets. Local government plays a minor role and has only limited tasks in the area of long-term care provision. However, local government is becoming more active in coordinating housing and care facilities for older people. It is likely that the influence of local municipalities will grow as they increasingly act in coordination with regional health authorities (the outposts of the national healthcare board). However, it is still very uncertain whether this increased regional–local cooperation will lead to greater decentralisation and local flexibility in the delivery of services and facilities, on the basis of an integrated 'regional budget'.

Second, public funding through the national healthcare insurance fund continues to finance the provision of services by non-profit organisations and the relatively high levels of public service utilisation by older people. Apart from the well-known interplay of formal and informal care, the concepts of 'welfare pluralism' and the 'mixed economy of care' have not materialised in changes in the funding of long-term care services. However, it is possible that middle and higher income groups may begin to opt for private long-term care insurance cover, partly in response to the widespread introduction of service charges which are strongly related to personal income levels, partly facilitated by plans to introduce tax-deductible care insurance premiums, and – most important – partly because of changes in the social composition of emerging cohorts of older people with higher pensions, higher expectations and better health status.

Third, services are provided by private non-profit providers, who have to comply with general quality standards. Increasingly, local or regional providers of home care, residential care or nursing home services are building joint ventures and other alliances, and this is contributing to the emergence of an oligopolistic market. In response, central government is attempting to limit the negative side-effects of these alliances by introducing 'benchmarking' which will control service providers' outputs, quality, and prices through inter-provider comparisons of clearly defined 'products'.

Fourth, despite pressure from organisations representing disabled and older service users to extend the small experimental scheme which gives help in the form of cash benefits or 'personal budgets', an estimated 95% of all expenditure on long-term care provision still goes on services in kind. Policy makers are reluctant to respond to pressure to extend the 'personal budget' scheme, citing financial arguments (problems of cost containment), social reasons (problems relating to the employment rights of professional care-givers), and implementation problems (the difficulty of attuning personal budgets to accurate assessments of an individual's health problems, impairments and disabilities).

Overall, Dutch society has succeeded in maintaining relatively high levels of publicly-funded long-term care services, well targeted at those groups who are most in need of formal support. As in other countries, the system is coming under pressure from a number of different perspectives, including policy makers who emphasise the increasing importance of accountability and the promotion of cost-effectiveness, and user organisations who argue for greater flexibility in the composition of care arrangements and more freedom of choice in the selection of providers.

Increasing coordination: the development of integrated long-term care

The need for better coordination

As in other countries, the Dutch system of long-term care has been criticised for a persistent lack of coordination. At national government level, there is a lack of coherence in the planning and financing of interdependent services, which can prevent the development of innovative and more efficient care arrangements (Petersen and White, 1989). Among providers, the problem is the lack of systematical collaboration through interorganisational networks; this hampers the development of joint programmes targeted at clients with complex or multiple problems (Alter and Hage, 1993). At the service user level, these problems are manifest in older people receiving services which are inappropriate for their current needs (for example, blocking beds in hospitals); and in the failure to provide appropriate combinations of services for older people with multiple problems (Baldock and Evers, 1991b).

These coordination problems have been investigated at the level of local or regional networks of providers – hospitals, institutional care, community-based services, special housing and housing facilities (Coolen, 1997). The research distinguished between coordination at organisational and managerial levels in the planning of services and facilities, the development of new programmes and the allocation of resources, and coordination at operational levels, in responding to the complex needs and demands of individual clients. The study found that patterns of coordination resembled a loosely structured configuration, founded predominantly on informal communication and unstable coalitions based upon a temporary congruence of interests. In general, coordination at the operational levels of interprofessional communication was much better developed than at managerial levels, despite the fact that the latter was necessary for the successful implementation of innovative care arrangements which crossed the boundaries of different services such as institutional and community care, sheltered housing and long-term care. In addition, most networks tended towards segmentation, so that relatively high levels of social cohesion within service subsystems (such as community services, for instance) contrasted with the much poorer coordination between the different subsystems. For example, there is little coordination between adapted housing and long-term care provision, either at the level of national public policy or between the management of the various provider organisations, although there are now plans to improve this relationship.

Policy experiments

In most regions, central and local governments are trying to introduce greater coherence into services for high-risk groups such as chronically ill people, disabled people and frail older people. Two trends are identifiable: the introduction of new coordination mechanisms in service delivery systems, such as joint needs assessment, monitoring systems and case management; and the development of regional network organisations with responsibility for planning services, allocating resources and regulating service delivery. Evaluation of the latter development (Coolen, 1993; 1994) has indicated a positive impact on the quality of care, as indicated by client monitoring systems, better matching of demand and supply and, to a lesser extent, improved efficiency in care services.

Several local experiments have aimed at creating new organisational arrangements between long-term care providers. Key elements of these new structures are:

- an umbrella organisation formed from the providers of home care, voluntary help, residential homes, nursing homes and sheltered housing, operating as an authoritative decision-making structure;
- the planning of services and service delivery carried out within the framework of an integrated budget, which combines the resources available to the separate care providers;
- resources and personnel reallocated between services in response to changing demands from older people;
- community-based services organised into district teams which operate at the level of an urban neighbourhood or a rural village; residential and nursing homes brought together in an integrated regime;
- needs assessment to take a comprehensive, holistic approach; opportunities for community-based service interventions to be maximised, in order to reduce admissions to institutional care.

Evaluation of integrated long-term care initiatives

The strategy of building integrated service networks was sponsored by both the national government and the national health authority. Initially (1988-92) it formed part of a policy of substituting community-based services for institutional care. More recently (particularly from 1997) it has formed part of a strategy of increasing the effectiveness and diversity of service provision for an increasingly heterogeneous older population (Coolen, 1994; 1997). What consequences were observed, especially in the local or regional projects, which successfully integrated the planning and funding of long-term care as well as needs assessment and service delivery?

Many projects demonstrated that it was feasible to develop coordinated networks of providers. The coordinating or umbrella organisations of these networks were able to develop flexible care arrangements within the context of a regional budget, were able to demonstrate efficiency in their allocation of resources and were able to be innovative in response to the changing demands and preferences of clients.

Evaluations of these integrated care strategies (Coolen, 1994; Kraan et al, 1991) demonstrated a number of positive consequences. The projects improved the matching of demand and supply. By and large, they were able to meet the predominant preferences for community-based services and to improve the flexibility of service delivery. Older people with complex problems received better quality and better coordinated services and therefore expressed higher levels of client satisfaction. The projects offered greater opportunities for frail older people to maintain an independent lifestyle; this was reflected in a substantial reduction in rates of admission to institutional facilities. Informal care-givers continued to play an important role, despite the overall extension of community services. Finally, a number of the projects demonstrated increased cost-effectiveness in long-term care for elderly people, in that the coverage and/or the quality of care was improved while the total costs of services for a given population of older people stayed constant or were reduced.

These findings suggest that strategies of integrated long-term care can enhance the effectiveness of care, because they reduce the number of boundaries which impede the development of more flexible and responsive services. Secondly they can to some extent improve the efficiency of care services, because they create more incentives to develop innovative, cost-effective responses to complex or chronic care problems. In summary, improving quality and containing costs need not be contradictory objectives.

Increasing choice: personal service budgets for older people

Home care provision

The regular service providers in The Netherlands occupy a stable position in the care market. Facing little competition, they receive a yearly budget from the national care fund in exchange for agreed levels of activity in the provision of home care, nursing homes, residential homes and intermediate care services.

Home care providers in particular have developed a monopolistic structure as an intended consequence of central government's policies of rewarding 'economies of scale'. On average, a healthcare region (covering approximately 500,000 inhabitants) will have at most only a few certified home care provider organisations. These provide nearly all publicly-funded professional home help and home nursing services. Few commercial, for-profit providers have entered the market of home care; their small market share is restricted to more affluent older people.

In the near future, some changes in this situation are anticipated, as a result of the introduction of 'personal budgets' which enable service users to select the providers they prefer.

Despite high levels of satisfaction among service users, the standard home care provider organisations have come under severe criticism from interest groups of clients and other 'stakeholders', such as hospital managers and health insurance companies. Home care services have been accused of being inflexible and inefficient. Individual older people often receive care from a number of different employees from the same provider organisation, which creates coordination problems. Organisations of disabled people, in particular, have promoted the introduction of personal budgets, on the grounds that this can give service users greater freedom of choice over the type and frequency of the services they receive.

In contrast, opposition has come from the provider organisations, worried about the threat to their market share, and from trades unions concerned about the rights and entitlements of employees. The national board for long-term care also expressed anxieties about possible cost escalation.

Experimental phase

After some years of policy debate, an experiment to give older people personal budgets for home care services began in 1991. This experimental status was considered necessary because opinions were so deeply divided.

With their personal budgets, older people mainly purchase home help services from sector organisations, but are more likely to purchase home nursing from the established provider organisations. Evaluation of the experiment demonstrated that participants were very positive about their increased freedom of choice, about the control they had over how and by whom care was delivered and about a number of aspects of the quality of the care they received (Ramakers and Miltenburg, 1993).

National regulation of personal budgets

Following the positive outcome of the experiment, in 1994 the Health Insurance Fund Council produced guidelines for the introduction of a national regulation on personal budgets. These guidelines aim to prevent socially undesirable consequences, such as spending personal budget money on items for private consumption rather than care services, or employing care-givers outside of general labour market regulations. The regulation was introduced in 1995 (Ziekenfondsraad, 1995) and amended in 1996. Currently, personal budgets can be allocated to "persons in need of home nursing and/or home help services", so long as this need is expected to last longer than three months and clients will continue to live in their own home. The personal budget can be used to purchase professional help from established home care organisations or new providers. It can also be used to contract with and pay informal care-givers.

Eligibility for a personal budget depends upon an assessment of needs, taking into account what immediate family members can contribute to the support of the older person. The personal budget is calculated by multiplying the number of hours of care the older person is assessed to need by the registered price per hour of the indicated type of service. A reassessment of need is required every six months. Depending on the older person's personal income, they will be charged user fees similar to those charged for services in kind.

Apart from a small fixed sum of Dfl 2,400 per year (which can be spent on care entirely at the older person's discretion), the older person is not actually in direct control of their personal budget. An Association of Personal Budget Holders acts as an intermediary between the client and the provider organisation. This arrangement was negotiated with the Ministries of Social Affairs and Finance because of anxiety about the possible purchase of care services in the 'grey', or unofficial, labour market and the consequent evasion of care workers' social security contributions and income taxes. The Association is responsible for paying the service providers (including the social security contributions and taxes of care workers). The user remains in control of the selection of providers, but delegates most of the financial administration of the personal budget to the Association. (From the beginning of 1998, these responsibilities of the Association of Personal Budget Holders were transferred to a branch of social security administration.)

Under the personal budget regime, both the established non-profit provider organisations and the new for-profit providers can deliver services. It is likely that the new for-profit provider organisations have a somewhat different clientele, who need fewer short-term interventions each day. This enables costs to be held down and maintains competitiveness with the established provider organisations in terms of price per average unit of service. Although some of the established provider organisations have complained of unfair competition, the empirical evidence is far from clear.

Both types of provider organisations have to meet three requirements: they must provide a broad range of services, including community nursing, help with activities of daily living, home help and the loan of technical equipment; they must comply with a single set of quality standards (mainly measured in terms of qualified personnel); and they must uphold collective labour agreements for professional home helpers and nursing personnel in home care (Boot and Knapen, 1996).

Uncertainty on the part of central government about the implications of the personal budget experiment means that it has so far been implemented only on a small scale; only 3% to 5% of the total care budget is currently spent in the form of personal budgets. For the year 1998, the overall budget for personal budgets has been set at 130 million Dutch guilders. Waiting lists for personal budgets are therefore common; if the annual macro-budget has already been spent, older people wishing to receive a personal budget receive services in kind while they wait. This restricted budget also limits the extent to which the current oligopolistic (sometimes monopolistic) structure of provider organisations might be transformed into a more competitive long-term care market. Managed competition has not really materialised in The Netherlands, reflecting widespread scepticism about the assumed advantages of privatising long-term care provision for older and disabled people. However, if the personal budget scheme was substantially extended, this would probably lead to a substantial shift in the social care market, with a reduced market share for the established home care agencies.

How older people use personal budgets

The services which older people buy with their personal budgets has been monitored regularly since the introduction of the scheme (Miltenburg and Ramakers, 1996a; 1996b; Ramakers and Miltenburg, 1997). The vast majority of beneficiaries are very positive about the opportunity to decide for themselves what care they want to buy, when and from whom. The main complaints have been about the lengthy and bureaucratic procedures for processing applications and inadequate information about entitlement and eligibility criteria. The average budget per client was about Dfl 1,500 per month. In 1997, approximately 5,500 people were allocated personal budgets.

Most recipients (54%) use the personal budget for domestic help only, 14% use their budget for personal or nursing care and 32% of recipients use the budget for a combination of services. This pattern of use more or less resembles the use of different long-term domiciliary care services among older people as a whole. Recipients allocate their budgets to a range of formal and informal care-givers. A third (37%) hire informal care-givers or private domestic help and two thirds (63%) contract with a professional agency (non-profit or for-profit, although the latter has the larger market share of personal budget recipients). Some beneficiaries think of the personal budget primarily as a way of rewarding informal care-givers who have already been providing support over a long period.

Table 4.3: Types of home care services used by personal budget recipients (1997)

Type of home care	Percentage
Home nursing	4
Personal care (ADL)	10
Home help	54
A combination of various types of care	32
Total	**100**

According to clients, personal budgets have led to better services, more control over how the job is done and more choice over who provides the care. For example, clients can now dismiss an employee or provider organisation if they are not satisfied. The most striking finding from evaluation studies concerns the improved quality of services and feelings of autonomy experienced by older people:

> **With the personal budget I have a better grip on the care provided to me and they don't treat me as a number. When I received help from a regular home care organisation, I felt as though I was just a number to them. In those days the employees came at ever-varying hours and there was a great turnover. The workers I hire, based on my personal budget, usually come in time, and the agency no longer sends so many different ones. This way it is easier to form a bond with someone, and to trust someone completely. (Weekers and Pijl, 1998, p 171)**

In conclusion, the personal budget scheme is positively valued by older people. Moreover, because of the safeguards built into the administration of the scheme, the risk of misuse is avoided. An indirect consequence is the increased pressure on established provider organisations to become more competitive in terms of quality and price, despite the very modest implementation of the scheme.

Independent living: housing and care

The impact of housing provision on demand for long-term care

Policy makers assume that adapted housing and access to neighbourhood facilities such as shops and public transport will help older people maintain an independent lifestyle and reduce demand for institutional care. This assumption has been tested empirically. Controlling for need variables, household and income, research has shown that adapted and sheltered housing schemes for older people do not reduce demands for institutional care. Moreover, people in adapted housing use more professional home care services than those living at home; this may reflect a 'reference group' effect, where older people living in close proximity together develop higher expectations of services. Deficiencies in the physical condition of the home are not correlated with the use of home care or demand for institutional care. Similarly, a lack of local amenities does not affect the use of home care services, though it does slightly increase demand for institutional care (Zijderveld-Blom and Coolen, 1992).

There are two possible reasons why special housing does not appear to reduce demand for institutional or home care services. First, local government and provider organisations have been somewhat cautious in their allocation of sheltered housing and have tended to admit less severely disabled older people (indeed, the levels of disability among residents of sheltered and adapted housing is similar to those of older people living in their own homes). Second, prevailing funding regimes do not allow for flexible service packages, over and above conventional home care services, which could enable very frail older people with little informal support to remain living in their own (adapted or sheltered) houses.

This shortcoming has prompted another new development. Conventional sheltered housing schemes designed in the 1970s consisted of technically adapted housing, with access to help from the staff of a local service centre or home for older people in the event of an emergency. However, since the late 1980s, extended sheltered housing schemes have been developed, involving collaboration between public housing corporations, home care provider organisations and local residential and nursing homes. In most projects, a case manager is appointed to arrange packages of services to meet the needs of older clients. If the health of an older client changes, the type and intensity of services can be altered without the older person having to be admitted to an institution.

Evaluation of extended sheltered housing initiatives

Although policy makers claim that these extended sheltered housing schemes function as fully fledged alternatives to institutional care, their cost-effectiveness is still being evaluated. So far, studies (Romijn et al, 1991) have demonstrated that extended sheltered housing can provide effective and flexible responses to the changing needs of older people with chronic health problems and reduce admissions to residential and nursing homes. They are also efficient, in that they offer care of the same quality as in institutional settings but at lower overall cost. Improvements in cost-effectiveness are most apparent among older people who might otherwise have entered residential care homes but lower among those with serious disabilities and dementia who might otherwise have entered nursing homes. Inputs of informal help remained more or less constant. There was a small improvement in the well-being of clients, but no significant reduction in the prevalence of reported loneliness.

Some projects indicated a tendency to create new demands for services, attracting a client group which was somewhat less frail and vulnerable than the intended target group of potential entrants to institutional care. These new clients tend to be from higher socioeconomic groups, which may reflect an emerging social stratification in long-term care for older people. Traditional institutional facilities are predominantly used by older people from lower social strata, whereas the new care arrangements, with their higher quality dwelling units, tend to attract more affluent older people who can afford the relatively higher costs.

Future trends

Long-term care in The Netherlands has elements of both continuity and change, within the context of a universalistic welfare state tradition. It remains centrally controlled and publicly-funded, with relatively high levels of service utilisation as an accepted outcome. However, a number of new developments are likely to dominate the political agenda in the imminent future.

First, there is likely to be greater decentralisation in the planning of long-term care within the framework of regionally integrated budgets formed from the national care insurance funds and resources from local governments. The regional authorities for long-term care (*Zorgkantoor*), acting together with local administrations, are under pressure to improve flexibility in service delivery. Managed care and benchmarking techniques will be used to improve the efficiency and effectiveness of providers in responding to the needs of older and disabled people.

Second, network arrangements between different long-term care service sectors are likely to increase, in order to improve service integration and reduce the boundaries between institutional and community-based care. These networks vary from the simple coordination of service delivery to the creation of integrated organisations which can deliver a flexible range of care arrangements across traditional boundaries of institutional and community care. These developments create new opportunities for delivering intensive care, similar to the level of services provided in residential and nursing homes, to very disabled older people in their own homes.

Third, it is likely that private markets for long-term care will continue to develop, following the growth in private care insurance schemes. This partly reflects the emergence of new cohorts of more affluent older people and partly the expansion of means-testing and income-related charges for publicly-funded services. This is part of a European-wide trend towards new social divisions in long-term care, in which private markets offer considerable consumer choice to higher income groups and publicly-funded care is increasingly restricted to cover the needs of only the poorer older people.

Achieving greater coordination

One of the most persistent criticisms of long-term care in The Netherlands has been its lack of flexibility. The care services which can be funded from public resources are strictly regulated by central government and the national board. These regulations implicitly reflect the notion of a hierarchical system of long-term care: community services for older people with manageable disabilities who can live in their own homes; sheltered housing for those with poorer health or who need extra support over and above the usual community services; and institutional care for those with multiple disabilities or psycho-geriatric disorders.

This segmentation creates recurring problems in assigning older people to the appropriate level of service provision and creates difficulties for service planners and policy makers in the numbers of older people receiving inappropriate services because of discrepancies between demand and supply or breakdowns in coordination across boundaries. However, these longstanding problems are being addressed through the concept of 'redesign' – replacing traditional divisions between services with 'packages' made up from a variety of services, which are allocated to older people on the basis of independent assessments. Thus care arrangements which are based on specific services provided by specific organisations will be replaced by programmes of services, tailored to specific client groups, and delivered by networks of provider organisations. In the next few years, this system redesign will probably be the most prevalent development in Dutch long-term care services.

At local and regional levels, provider networks will certainly develop, regardless of central government policy. Networked relationships between traditional providers of community services and institutional care will be able to establish greater control over the (publicly funded) market of long-term care, in opposition to new (for-profit) providers; they can expect to achieve some 'economies of scale' in the process and may also manage to avoid competition between providers in the 'zero-sum' situation of fixed budgets. The shift from institutional to community-based services, predominantly driven by the changing expectations and preferences of new cohorts of older people, can also be addressed by redirecting the resources of institutional providers through the means of a network organisation.

The future of personal budgets

A widespread extension of the personal budget scheme will probably not materialise during the next few years, because of the major implications this would have for the regulation of long-term care provision. It is also unlikely that entitlement to a personal budget will be placed on a statutory basis, similar to social security benefit entitlements. At present, if the total budget for personal budgets is exhausted, then an applicant who is otherwise entitled is simply placed on a waiting list.

The personal budget scheme will probably continue as it is today, involving only a small proportion of the macro-budget, giving some incentive to providers to enhance their responsiveness to clients, but without threatening the market position of the traditional non-profit organisations.

The Ministry of Finance has initiated a project to explore the feasibility of a (more universal) system of vouchers, instead of the current restricted personal budget scheme. Vouchers might provide an alternative means of exchange between an older person with care needs and certified provider organisations. The possible use of vouchers is partly seen as a means of providing greater flexibility over the choice of services for individual users and partly as a means of containing continuing pressures for increased funding for long-term care.

User control

A major problem remains the limited influence which clients are able to exercise over service provision. However, the national government has introduced regulations which facilitate the process of empowerment (for instance, a rule that every provider organisation must set up a board of user representatives). In addition, the government has enforced a policy of independent needs assessment, whereby (semi-)public agencies process requests for long-term care services and thus counterbalance the power of providers. This gatekeeping function may enhance consumer choice. However, the organisations carrying out the assessments will inevitably encounter the inherent tensions between rising expectations and demands and the restricted financial resources for long-term care.

FIVE

Community care for frail older people in Finland

Kristiina Martimo

Introduction

This chapter will describe the changes in funding arrangements between central and local government which were introduced in Finland in 1993, the slow development of integrated health and social services at municipal levels, the organisation of decision making and financial management of primary health services, the introduction of charges for health and welfare services, and changes in the system of care allowances.

In Finland, major changes in health and social services provision occurred after the economic recession of 1991. The recession was caused by the collapse of the Soviet Union, Finland's largest trading partner. In addition, serious problems within the money markets forced the government to use considerable amounts of public funds to rescue banks. During this profound economic recession, national unemployment rose to around 20% and a reassessment of welfare expenditure became essential.

At the same time, demographic changes in the population structure are placing increasing pressures on the financing of welfare and healthcare services for older people in Finland. Between 1990 and 2010 the number of people over 80 years old in Finland is expected to increase by about 200% (Vaarama, 1995). In contrast, in Sweden, England and Germany the numbers of over 80-year-olds will increase by only 50% (OECD, 1992, in Vaarama, 1995). After 2030 the increase in the numbers of very elderly people will slow down in Finland, because the number of over 80-year-olds will have reached its peak at the end of 2010. The main impact of these demographic changes will therefore occur between 2020 and 2030, when the numbers of very elderly people will be at their greatest (Heikkila, 1995):

> In the present economic crisis services for the elderly are changing. This involves on one hand using the shrinking resources better and on the other hand making changes so that the services can cope with the challenges of the next century. (Vaarama, 1995, p 18)

In all Scandinavian countries there is a strong tradition of local self-government. This is seen as a cornerstone of local democracy. Municipalities have the right to levy their own local taxes and local governments have a long history of providing a diverse range of social services (Kroger, 1997). In Scandinavia, the production of social care services rests upon a close alliance between local municipalities and the state. The government provides subsidies for locally organised services and national legislation obliges local municipalities to produce them. When the economy and the welfare state were growing, the national government specified and regulated the level of services which were expected to be provided by the municipalities. However, at present the municipalities have considerable autonomy in deciding what levels of service provision to offer (Sipilä, 1997).

Social welfare and healthcare services developed from the early 1980s and the municipalities were allocated new responsibilities by central government. In 1984 central government funding for the provision of social welfare services by the municipalities was increased to equal that for health services and research into the productivity and efficiency of municipalities was commissioned (Iivari, 1995). By the end of the 1980s, however, the relationship between central and local government began to come under scrutiny, with the municipalities pressing for greater local autonomy, and central government wanting less involvement in and responsibility for local affairs.

In Finland the private sector has not been a provider of welfare services to any significant degree. The larger cities have private hospitals, which are used by wealthier people in order to avoid waiting lists. Some leisure-related social welfare activities are provided by voluntary, religious, and charitable organisations. These services only constitute about 10% of total provision. However, the number of services for which charges are made has increased significantly since the reforms of 1993, which gave municipalities the freedom to charge for both health and social welfare services. According to the Social and Health Ministry, municipal expenditure on social welfare and healthcare should remain largely financed from taxation rather than user charges (Ministry of Social Affairs and Health, 1993). Overall, Finland still retains many features of the Scandinavian welfare state, with the majority of services collectively funded from central and local taxation and provided by local government organisations. However, both these traditions have been coming under increased pressures as the result of economic and demographic changes.

The importance of local variations

One of the difficulties in describing health and social care services for older people in Finland is the enormous variety of different ways of organising and providing services between 460 municipalities, which vary considerably in size and financial circumstances. Generalisation is difficult. For example, some municipalities offer most services free of charge and have strong organisational links to encourage cooperation between different service providers, while other municipalities provide few services and make charges for them. Even within the 25 largest municipalities, there are vast differences and variations in service provision for older people (Viialainen and Lehto, 1996). These local differences in social and health services funding, policies and organisation are so great that it is feasible to talk about different service cultures between municipalities (Vaarama, 1995).

The trend towards greater local autonomy

The history of the strong municipality started in Finland in the middle of the nineteenth century, when the municipalities broke away from church organisations to become the main unit of local government. Within this new separation between local civil and religious government, the municipalities took responsibility for poor relief.

Before this century, all the Scandinavian countries apart from Denmark were extremely poor. The first social care service – a children's day care centre for working class families – opened in Helsinki in 1888, with support from the city authorities (Sipilä, 1997). Legislation in the Scandinavian countries in the 1920s and 1930s led to the development of professional social welfare and healthcare services, not just for humanitarian reasons, but also to reduce the risk of social unrest (Sipilä, 1997).

The 'free municipality' experiment began in Finland in 1989 along lines developed in Sweden, which had first experimented with giving more autonomy to the municipalities. The aims were to simplify municipal and central government powers, and to increase the powers of the individual citizen by creating small area meetings which would decide on the service provision and structure for their local area. It was assumed that localising decisions about the provision of services to sub-municipality level would enable services to be more responsive and better targeted at the right service users. However, these small area meetings did not materialise and power has shifted to the municipal bureaucrats, who make the plans and present them to the municipal politicians (Paivarinta, private communication).

The 'free municipality' experiment helped to pave the way for major state subsidy changes in 1993. Pressure was also developing from within the municipalities, who were beginning to purchase services from voluntary and private sector providers as a way of introducing competition and reducing costs. In order to make this process more workable, the municipalities needed to be more autonomous and have greater control over the financing of the services they provided (Iivari, 1995).

Until 1993, central government funded around 50% of both sheltered housing for older people and residential care homes, the other 50% coming from the municipalities. Again up to 1993, central government also exercised considerable control over municipal social welfare and health services; central government monitored and regulated the service provision of the municipalities (Hutten and Kerkstra, 1996). The municipalities had to apply for central government subsidies, giving a detailed record of the services they would offer. They were also required to report back with detailed information on how service development plans had been implemented and whether cost forecasts had been adhered to.

In 1993 the state subsidy system was redeveloped and these tight central controls were relinquished. Central government subsidies specifically for particular social welfare and healthcare services ended and the levels of subsidies were no longer calculated according to the costs or the range of service provision. Now municipalities receive a single block grant from central government, which they are free to allocate as they wish (Sipilä and Anttonen, 1994). The block grant subsidy is calculated separately for each municipality according to a formula which takes into account the number of residents of different ages in the municipality, their wealth and morbidity. At the same time as this major change took place, the overall level of central government funding to the municipalities was cut. Central government justified these savings by arguing that the economies of many of the municipalities were in a far better condition than those of the Finnish state (Uusitalo, 1996).

Under the new system municipalities can decide which services they will provide, and also whether they will be provided through private care providers or through municipal organisations. Municipalities can, for instance, decide to give priority to primary and community health services and leave social care services with fewer resources. The only remaining element of central government regulation is in relation to capital investment, such as hospital or polyclinic construction.

This major change in relationships between central and local government and the greatly enhanced autonomy of the municipalities has left service users in a vulnerable position, because some municipalities may be unable to provide the full range of services, particularly while they are still suffering the consequences of economic recession (Hutten and Kerkstra, 1996). However, the change reflects a long political battle to give more power to local government:

> **The municipalities have also repeatedly used the principle of local self-government as the main legitimating source in their sharp criticism of those initiatives of the welfare state which have been aimed at broadening central regulation. (Kroger, 1997, p 101)**

Iivari (1995) argues that the major reason for reducing the power of central government lay in the growing confusion about the division of responsibilities between the two tiers of government. The relationship between the state and the municipalities had developed into a fragmented and divided system, so much so that the legislation governing the control by central government of municipal expenditure was beginning to be unworkable. The state subsidy system was complicated, heavy and cumbersome to operate. The severe recession of the early 1990s was also a major force in speeding up the drive for change, because the municipal economies were growing weaker by the end of the 1980s and this created a need for changes in the municipal budgeting structure (Iivari, 1995). The recession was at its deepest between 1992-93, and it was at this point that the fundamental changes were introduced in the legislation regulating central government's involvement in social welfare and healthcare planning and finance (Iivari, 1995).

The reorganisation of the municipal subsidy system had two aims: to strengthen the autonomy of the municipalities, thereby giving them greater responsibility over the allocation of their resources; and to diminish the role of central government in the regulation of municipal service provision.

Instead of central government retaining regulatory power over the budgets of the municipalities, the municipalities were given much greater freedom to determine their own spending priorities. Their responsibility to provide services remains intact, but the levels, organisation and quality of these services are now no longer prescribed by central government. Central government has also been able to distance itself from the political consequences of fiscal retrenchment. There has been some discussion recently of the need to reintroduce some regulation by central government in order to combat the regional inequalities in service provision which have now emerged (Paivarinta, private communication).

The organisation and funding of health and welfare services in Finland

The principles of the Finnish healthcare system are very similar to those of other European countries (Makela, 1996). Since 1972, the development of primary health services has been a major priority in Finnish health policy. Primary healthcare in the public sector is provided in community health centres, where preventive healthcare clinics are organised for people of different age groups and with different medical problems. Local health policy is decided by boards of publicly elected politicians. Some private sector primary health services are available, mainly through workplace-based healthcare facilities, private family practitioners and private health centres which are found in large cities.

Every municipality either has a health centre of its own or one which it shares with neighbouring municipalities. A large health centre serving 25,000 people will have a number of primary care teams, each of which includes a general practitioner, two or three health visitors or nurses and a secretary. Health centres also provide dental services, physiotherapy and diagnostic services and some beds for in-patient treatment. Since the early 1990s it is increasingly common to require patients to register with a physician before they can make an appointment to see any of the general practitioners working in the health centre. Many people see the 'own doctor' service as a positive development in primary care (Hanninen et al, 1995). More specialist secondary care is provided in regional hospitals, each providing services for a number of municipalities. Most people with chronic, relatively stable conditions will receive treatment in health centre beds rather than regional hospitals.

The municipalities receive between 30% and 65% of the total cost of the primary and secondary health services they provide from central government, depending on the size of their population and morbidity indicators. Users pay about 10% of the health service budget in the form of charges for services provided. The remainder is raised from local taxation. Again an uneven picture emerges, because in some municipalities charges are made for health centre visits and in others they are not; home nursing is charged for in some areas and not in others. Although health centre-based general practitioners are available for everyone in the area, in some municipalities the charging of fees for visits or treatment makes it difficult for some people to afford a visit to the doctor. War veterans and children under 15 are exempted from all of these charges.

Some services, such as private medical practice and dental care for adults, are funded entirely through user fees. The user is then entitled to a 40% refund from the state health insurance scheme on all expenses incurred in the use of private healthcare (apart from dental care). The Finnish state health insurance is compulsory and collected through taxation. In other words, taxpayers in Finland finance both public and private healthcare, through the health insurance scheme. This "is currently being strongly challenged in policy debates" (Makela, 1996, p 42).

The main primary healthcare services used by older people are GP services and visits to the health centre, with the most common consultation among the over 65s being for high blood pressure and diabetes. Home nursing is more widely used in Finland compared with the rest of Europe; it is mostly offered to people over 75 years of age in an effort to avoid hospitalisation (Raassina, 1994).

Both health and welfare services are planned and organised by the municipalities. As well as GP services, home nursing and some beds in health centres, health services also include long-term institutional care and services for younger and older people with mental health problems. Social welfare services include home help, other support services (meals on wheels, transport, sauna and bathing, laundry and security services), day centres, sheltered housing and residential care homes. Municipalities also provide care allowances in lieu of services, to support the home care of some frail older people (see below).

Finland has, until very recently, provided a considerable volume of public sector institutional care for older people, either in health centre hospitals as part of local primary health services or in residential care homes which are run by municipal social welfare departments. Since the 1970s, the number of institutional places for older people has decreased, despite the increase in the numbers of very elderly people. In 1984, major welfare reforms took place and funding for social welfare services for older people was increased, to reduce the reliance of municipalities on more expensive health-based care services:

> **The trend was to harmonise state subsidies to different sectors of social welfare and to raise them to the same level as in healthcare. The idea was to develop social care services instead of the more expensive healthcare services, especially for the elderly. (Sipilä, 1997, p 34)**

The fastest growing elements of social welfare services for older people are the home help and domiciliary support services. During the 1980s, these grew faster in Finland than in other Scandinavian countries (Raassina, 1994). In 1992, about 8% of the total municipal social welfare budgets went on home help and support services. One in five of all over 65-year-olds receives home help and support services, which makes Finland one of the most generous countries in providing these services (Raassina, 1994). A study of satisfaction with municipalities' service provision found that only 6% of respondents thought they did not receive enough help at home (Viialainen and Lehto, 1996). Finnish home helps are a quasi-professional group. Their training involves a full-time two-and-a-half year course and most are employed on a full-time basis.

However, in areas with fewer older people or with high numbers of hospital beds, municipalities still use hospital beds instead of home helps and domiciliary support services. Particularly in the north of Finland, where long distances create major problems in delivering domiciliary services, it is more economical to provide long-term institutional care instead of domiciliary social welfare services, a care allowance, a home help or support services. There may be limits, therefore, in these municipalities in the extent to which the staff of institutional services can be transferred to primary and home care services.

Integration of social welfare and health services

> **The collaboration between primary care and the social services is a very important development.... Team work development and the care of the elderly are real challenges where this collaboration is helpful. (Makela, 1996, p 45)**

Although both health and social welfare services are organised by the municipalities, the degree of coordination between them is highly variable.

In some municipalities, the different services are in close contact, whereas in others there is little collaboration.

The integration of municipal social welfare and primary and community health services began in some municipalities in the 1970s. In the 1980s only a few municipalities had combined the administration of social welfare and healthcare but by 1994 almost 40% of the population lived in municipalities in which healthcare and social services are part of the same organisation. Although this does not necessarily mean that social and health services are fully integrated, increasing numbers of municipalities are now running combined health and social care centres. Moreover, there are moves to extend the principle of 'small area responsibility', to replace the traditional separate organisations for different types of services. The functions of health and social care centres may extend further in the future, to include home nursing and home help services, housing and environmental services.

However, in order to achieve economies of scale, many small municipalities have joined together in small 'federations' and pooled the funding and administration of their primary care health centre facilities. This will prevent the full integration of social welfare and health administration in the smaller municipalities (Lehto and Vaarama, 1996).

During the recession of the early 1990s, the integration of health and social services was identified as one of the ways to make savings and improve services, especially in relation to the coordination of home care services and home nursing. Welfare and health services operating in isolation without any sharing of information about each other's workload risk duplicating services, particularly in larger municipalities where there are fewer opportunities for informal, face to face contacts between professional staff. In addition, separate sectors can shift costs to each other by cutting their own service provision (Vaarama, 1995).

Melin (1995) examined 11 different municipalities and the services they offer to older people, focusing on their efforts to combine social welfare and healthcare, flexibility of staff and the overall aims of the services for older people in different municipalities. The municipalities were divided into high and low spending ones. The high spending municipalities received higher central government subsidies and their older people lived in poorer conditions (as indicated, for example, in high levels of poor quality or inappropriate housing). However, the services for older people in these municipalities were also less efficient and cost-effective, because these municipalities also tended to offer high levels of institutional, rather than community-based services. This was because of the investment which had already been made in the physical fabric and staffing of long-stay hospital services and the difficulty of switching funding to invest in training staff to provide home-based services.

Most of the high spending municipalities were in the north of Finland, where the population is sparse and distances between shops, hospitals, health centres and settlements are very great. Here the living conditions of older people also tend to be poorer. Distance clearly adds to the costs of domiciliary services and makes their provision more difficult (Kroger, private communication). It also creates difficulties in coordinating the planning and delivery of services for such a dispersed population.

Low spending municipalities, on the other hand, had higher proportions of older residents with better living conditions and better health than high spending municipalities. The low spending municipalities also had strong commitments to developing services for older people and long traditions of both service development work and collaboration.

The low spending municipalities had taken a more proactive and positive approach to the cuts and reorganisation of the central government subsidies in 1993. They saw the new block grant subsidy system as offering greater flexibility to target services and improve cost-effectiveness. However, the single block grant subsidy did create problems, particularly in relation to the development of social welfare services. The demands of the health sector (particularly specialist hospital services) tended to take priority over social welfare services; this also made it difficult to move resources from medical and institutional care facilities into home and community-based services.

The continuing economic problems in Finland may threaten the further integration of health and social welfare services, because of a shortage of resources to finance organisational changes. However, effective cooperation has been shown to cut costs and increase efficiency, for example, by eliminating duplication between home help and home nursing services. Improved coordination and cooperation, particularly between health and social welfare services, has been shown to be associated with efficiency and lower levels of expenditure (Vaarama, 1995). In contrast, high spending, lower performing municipalities tend to have higher levels of collaboration between municipal social welfare services and church and voluntary organisations, rather than health.

Charging for services

The 1993 subsidy changes were accompanied by new permissive powers which now allow municipalities to make charges for the services they provide. However, the Finance Committee of the Social and Health Ministry (Karjalainen, 1994) recommended that the costs of services should not have a negative impact on users' standards of living, that charges should not exceed a maximum yearly fee (except for long-term institutional care) and that the levels of charges should take into account the income and assets of individual service users. These recommendations covered only charges for municipal services; the charges levied by voluntary organisations offering specialist services like sheltered housing are not controlled (Paivarinta, private communication).

There are major variations between municipalities in the extent to which they have taken advantage of this new freedom, the services for which they now make charges and the levels of charges they impose. For example, some municipalities charge for visits to the doctor, but others consider that the collection of such charges costs more than the revenue generated from the fees. Because of these variations, it is impossible to make any generalisation about the costs of services to users, because these will depend on the area they live in.

The Social and Health Ministry Finance Committee's 1993 report recommended that municipal social and healthcare services should remain predominantly tax financed. However, in the long term it is planned to increase charges for services in social welfare by up to 30% to 40% and in healthcare by 20%, and to extend charges to all services except health promotion. Currently, municipalities are tending to increase charges for home care services (Vaarama and Hurskanen, 1993); this trend is likely to continue, with higher charges being made for social welfare services than for healthcare (with the exception of long-term institutional care). This, argue Vaarama and Hurskanen (1993), demonstrates the dominance of the medical model in services for older people.

Monthly charges for regular home support services were introduced in 1993 (Raassina, 1994); this led to a decrease in demand for these services (Sipilä, 1997). Charges for home care services vary between municipalities. Some municipalities charge according to the length of the visit and clients' income, some on just the length of the visit, while others have a flat rate for everyone. Most municipalities have extended both the range of services for which charges are made and the range of clients who are now affected (Karjalainen, 1994). Cleaning, for instance, can cost from 20 FMK to 80 FMK (between £2.50 and £10) an hour, depending on where the older person lives (Karjalainen, 1994). Indeed, many municipalities are trying to move away from providing cleaning services by effectively pricing themselves out of the market (Kroger, private communication).

In recent years in Finland, there has been debate about the introduction of a voucher system to pay for some welfare services (Raassina, 1994). Vouchers would increase the range of providers and hence users' ability to choose between service providers; they also provide an effective means of controlling demand for services. Vouchers are seen as working best in services which do not require much training, such as the provision of meals and cleaning. The introduction of vouchers would require explicit criteria as to who is eligible, mechanisms for monitoring the quality of services and the provision of information to service users about the quality of services available. In addition, basic services would still have to be guaranteed to those older people who do not want to use vouchers or cannot do so (Raassina, 1994). So far there is little experience in the use of the voucher systems for services, although some municipalities began to introduce them in the spring of 1995 (Lehto and Vaarama, 1996).

Care allowances after recent changes

An established feature of social welfare provision in Finland, both in relation to the home care of older people and day care for young children, is the provision of cash allowances instead of services in kind (Glendinning and McLaughlin, 1993a; 1993b). Allowances are provided in respect of the care needs of the older person, but are paid by the municipality directly to a carer (who does not necessarily have to be a family member or share the household of the older person). The carer enters into a contract with the municipality to provide an agreed level of care to the older person in return for the allowance. Care allowances provide a viable alternative to the provision of the very intensive home care services which would be needed to keep a very frail older person out of institutional care, but which would be particularly difficult to provide in sparsely populated areas. Moreover, they are effective in capping expenditure on long-term care services. Even for people with very high care needs who require round-the-clock attention, a care allowance is considerably lower than the cost of providing the professional home help and home support services which would be needed (Glendinning and McLaughlin, 1993b).

The level of care allowances varies very considerably between municipalities. In 1993 legislative amendments established a minimum level for the allowance. Concern had previously been expressed at the lack of practical support available to carers and older people who received care allowances; municipal social welfare departments rarely followed up care allowance recipients to assess their continued ability to provide care (Glendinning and McLaughlin, 1993a). The 1993 changes therefore introduced an option whereby part of the care allowance can be provided in the form of support services, the total value of this cash and care package not exceeding the level of the care allowance.

In 1994, 394 out of 402 municipalities (92%) paid care allowances (Antikainen and Vaarama, 1995). Around 13,000 disabled and elderly people received a home care allowance, two thirds of them being over 65 years old. Without the allowance, two thirds of recipients would have had to enter long-term institutional care. Of the carers, 31% were spouses, 64% other relatives and the rest were unrelated. Most carers were over 50 years old and a third were over 65. Around 25% of recipients received part of their care allowance in the form of home support services. The average monthly allowance was approximately 1,496 FMK, with variations between 250 and 5,500 FMK a month. In about half the municipalities, the carer's own income level affected the level of the allowance, with poorer carers receiving higher level allowances. A third of municipalities – mainly those in sparsely populated rural areas where older people's living conditions are poorer – took the economic situation of the older person into account in assessments for care allowances (Antikainen and Vaarama, 1995).

Increasingly stringent means-testing in some municipalities has increased the targeting of the allowance on the poorest older people and carers and also reduced the overall numbers of care allowance recipients.

Assessments and the allocation of care allowances are carried out differently in different municipalities. Home care coordinators, social workers and managers, managers of old people's homes and members of social welfare boards (or any combination of these) can be involved (Antikainen and Vaarama, 1995). From 1993, municipalities have also been required to arrange time off for carers who have contracted with them to provide care. However, only a third of municipalities arrange time off for carers as required by law.

It could be argued that care allowances are an excellent example of the regional variations which permeate the whole service provision for older people. The amount of money paid for heavy care work varied almost six-fold between different municipalities in 1994 (Antikainen and Vaarama, 1995).

Outcomes

The present generation of frail older people in Finland is used to self-reliance and harsh living conditions during and after the war. Because of this, their expectations of welfare services are relatively low. Services for older people were not an issue at the last local elections; the only forum for discussions about regional differences and variations in service provision for older people are in academic circles. However, it may be that the next generation of older people and their children will bring these issues to the top of the social policy agenda and demand more equality and quality control in the service provision of primary healthcare and social welfare for frail older people.

Despite the recent debates about the possible introduction of vouchers, which might imply an intention of increasing choice for service users, there has been relatively little development of alternative private sector welfare provision. The only services in which any alternatives to municipal suppliers have developed are occupation-related healthcare facilities and the provision of traditional home help, domestic cleaning services, in which many municipalities are now trying to reduce their role.

At present, Finland seems like a large laboratory of social welfare and healthcare provision, with a number of different strategies for service provision in operation. However, there has been discussion and debate recently about the need to increase once again the regulatory role of central government, in order to reduce the very high levels of inequality and variability currently apparent in both social welfare and healthcare provision (Paivarinta, private communication). However, it is easy to overstate the significance of the 1993 subsidy changes in this respect. Municipalities have always had very high levels of autonomy in deciding what levels of services to provide, for whom and at what charges, in order to fulfil their basic obligation to provide 'enough' services to meet 'local needs'. Older people who are registered disabled do have entitlements to services such as transport, sheltered housing and home support services, but this has not prevented some municipalities from withdrawing services such as transport altogether because of economic problems. There are currently a number of legal test cases challenging these developments and seeking to strengthen the legal rights of disabled older people (Kroger, private communication).

The main significance of the 1993 subsidy changes may, in the long term, lie in the potential offered to municipalities to make radical changes in the balance and patterns of services, to shift resources from high cost institutional care, for example, and increase opportunities for service substitution and to reduce duplication between services. Many municipalities face major obstacles in realising this potential, because of their large distances, sparse populations, fragile local economies and relatively poor older people. Even so, research evidence suggests considerable diversity between municipalities in the extent to which they have responded to these new challenges.

SIX

Health and social care for older people in Denmark: a public solution under threat?

Lone Lund Pedersen

Introduction

Care for older people in Denmark has been in transformation since the beginning of the 1980s. In the 1980s the whole policy mood was characterised by the spirit of de-institutionalisation. This policy, termed 'in own home for as long as possible', sought to replace nursing home care with a network of services to keep people in their homes or in purpose built accommodation. The 1980s also saw the closure of beds for older people in both somatic and psychiatric hospitals and trends towards reduced lengths of stay and earlier discharge of older people (Alban et al, 1988). De-institutionalisation was based on an expectation of economic savings as well as philosophies of enhancing self-realisation, increased choice and autonomy, which had been identified as central objectives by the Elder Commission (1982). The Elder Commission was established in 1979 by the Minister of Social Affairs with a remit to assess the conditions of older people and propose ways in which to improve these. It was very influential in shaping subsequent service developments and policies, not least with respect to coordinated service provision, which took up a whole volume of its three volume report (Elder Commission, 1980; 1981; 1982). With the move to care in the community, significant changes in the organisation of community care services followed. However, the policy also raised concerns about the extent to which it revealed gaps in community care services, and about the impact of the policy on the overall coherence and continuity of care for older people who needed hospital care.

In the 1990s the agenda has, as in many other European countries, been dominated by increasing pressures on the public sector resulting from demographic changes and from expenditure limits imposed by economic harmonisation in the EU and declining public support for increasing taxes (Ministry of Finance, 1995). A further pressure has been the changing composition of the population of older people, with an increasing number of younger, resourceful and more critical older people who are demanding better services. In Denmark the response to this debate has been for public authorities to seek new types of both health and social care services and new ways of increasing efficiency. These have included increasing the involvement of non-public, voluntary sector organisations in service provision, and moves to increase efficiency, choice and competition by contracting out services from the public to the private sector.

This chapter examines these changes in greater detail. It is organised around the three dominant themes in the Danish policy for older people over the last 10 to 15 years. The following section describes the basic funding and structure of health and social welfare services in Denmark. The next section focuses on the de-institutionalisation policy and the associated creation of alternative forms of care in the community and changes in the organisation of this provision for older people. The chapter then focuses on the interface between hospital care and care in the community and issues of coordination. The final section discusses the issues surrounding the transfer of service provision from public to non-public sectors. The chapter concludes with an assessment of the consequences of these changes and their impact on the access to care and quality of care received by older people.

Denmark represents an example of what can be achieved within the parameters of publicly-funded health and social care services, in terms of quality of life and access to services for older people. The question is whether these qualities can be maintained in the future or whether it is a public solution under threat.

Organisation and funding of health and social services in Denmark

Two features characterise the Danish welfare state. One is the principle of universal, comprehensive and tax-financed welfare services. The other is a high degree of decentralisation in both decision-making powers and the financing of health and social services.

The first principle has three elements. First, compared with other modern welfare states, the Danish welfare state has retained a commitment to extensive public provision, including both generous universal income transfers and also a wide range of welfare services. It is an institutional welfare state. Second, these welfare services are either free or heavily subsidised. Third, the benefits are tax-financed rather than financed, for example, through labour market contributions or subscriptions from employers and protected persons. This means that all citizens are entitled not only to some form of income to replace lost earnings, but also to a comprehensive package of (largely) free health and social services when needed, regardless of labour market affiliation and to a large extent also regardless of income.

Public administration is divided into three levels: parliament and central government, which serves an overall population of just over 5 million people; 14 counties (with an average population of 295,000 inhabitants varying from 46,000 to 600,000); and 275 municipalities (with an average population of 19,000 inhabitants varying from 2,400 to 467,000 in the capital) (National Association of Municipalities, 1997). These three tiers constitute politically and administratively independent units. Both counties and municipalities have their own administrations and are headed by locally elected councils (*Kommunalbestyrelser*). Each of the three levels has specific tasks allocated on the basis of the subsidiarity principle. Counties and municipalities have a high degree of autonomy in decision making and in the organisation and financing of services. The latter area of autonomy includes the right to collect taxes and to determine the level of regional or local taxation[1]. Further financial decentralisation has taken place by largely replacing the previous reimbursement system by government block grants which, together with revenues from local taxation, constitute the financial basis for local services.

This second feature of the Danish welfare state is embodied in the principle of 'self-governing local councils' (*kommunalt selvstyre*). Responsibility for both health and social care services is fully delegated to local levels. Central government and parliament provide the legislative framework for both social and health services but the administration and implementation of provision are carried out at the two levels of local government. The main regulatory mechanism is the annual budget negotiations which take place at national level between the Ministry of Finance and the National Association of Municipalities (KL) – the collective body of the 275 municipalities. These negotiations set the municipalities' expenditure in the coming financial year, including limits on the rates of increase in expenditure and local taxation and agreements about special grants for areas of national priority. The option of setting minimum standards via national legislation as an additional regulatory mechanism is rarely used, because the introduction of any minimum standards which exceeded current service levels in the municipalities would prompt demands for special funding and would therefore have implications for the national budget.

Health and social services

In health and social care the Ministry of Health and the Ministry of Social Affairs provide the overall framework, setting out and allocating responsibilities between tiers of local government. Individual municipalities and county councils decide on the specific composition of local service packages. Broadly speaking, health and social care is divided into secondary care (hospitals), primary medical care (general practitioners and community-based specialist clinics) and other primary healthcare in the community (including nursing homes, community nursing and home help services). All medical healthcare services are the responsibility of the 14 counties, while non-medical community care is the responsibility of the 275 municipalities. Thus, both primary medical care and hospital care are fully operated by the counties and paid for from regional budgets. General practitioners are independent contractors working within a framework negotiated between medical doctors' organisations and the Association of County Councils (Platz and Petersen, 1992). They are remunerated by the National Health Insurance Scheme through a mixture of capitation and fee-for-service (Wagner, 1989; 1997). Hospitals are directly administered units, albeit with a high degree of autonomy. Both primary medical care and hospital care are provided free of charge (other services such as dentists and pharmacy are subsidised but involve a payment).

The municipalities are responsible for institutional and home care services, specialised housing for older people and a range of other services designed to help older people remain in their own homes for as long as possible. Nursing homes are the main form of institutional care provided by municipalities. They provide a total package of services including accommodation, nursing care and a range of additional services such as meals, practical assistance, cleaning, practical equipment, hairdressing, pedicure, therapy and leisure activities. Residents pay by contributing their full pension received from the state plus 60% of other income (Platz and Petersen, 1992; Boll Hansen, 1997).

The core domiciliary care services are home nursing and home help, both of which are provided free of charge. Both have to be provided by fully trained staff. Home nursing is usually short-term assistance with treatments such as dispensing medicine and changing catheters. Home help services assist with practical domestic tasks such as cleaning, cooking, laundry and shopping and personal care such as getting in and out of bed, dressing and hygiene (Plovsing, 1992; Danish Nurses' Organisation, 1989; 1991).

An important and integral aspect of local authority provision for older people in the community is special housing. A new type of housing was introduced in 1988 to replace nursing homes and older forms of municipal housing (sheltered housing, service flats and municipal pensioners' flats). Special housing consists of flats specifically adapted for the needs of older people. Some have staff and services attached, but the intention is to separate fully housing and care; when home care or nursing are needed they are provided by the municipalities' domiciliary care services. This idea derived from experiments in the early 1980s which were supported by the Minister of Social Affairs. Tenants of special housing pay rent according to their income – normally 15% – plus heating and electricity (Platz and Petersen, 1992; Boll Hansen, 1997).

Other services developed in the 1980s and 1990s in response to the 'in own home policy' (see below) include day centres and day care in nursing homes. In some municipalities, centres for older people have been built which provide opportunities for therapy and social activities; other municipalities have built pensioners' centres which are allocated to and run by older people themselves (Platz and Petersen, 1992). Older people living in their own homes may be offered transport to these centres. Other municipal services can include meals on wheels, help with gardening, snow clearance and other special services which are provided for a fee. Municipalities also loan out technical equipment and appliances and fund home improvements free of charge. There may also be access to emergency help via alarm systems (Boll Hansen, 1997).

Not only are health and social and community care services both public responsibilities, but responsibility for all non-medical long-term care in the community – including home nursing and home help services – is under the same tier of local government. This is the key to understanding the Danish case.

In sum, the 'package' of health and social services which older people are entitled to is quite comprehensive, particularly with respect to the community-based services administered and financed by the 275 municipalities. As with health services, most of these are provided free of charge, the exceptions being nursing home places, specialised housing and some extra practical services such as chiropody and hairdresssing.

The above describes current service arrangements. However, the range of services and the balance between them have been changing with the implementation of the 'as long as possible in own home policy' which is described below.

Access to services

Although services are allocated at the discretion of individual municipalities, in practice the allocation is actually very uniform across municipalities (Boll Hansen and Platz, 1995b). All community care services (nursing home places, home help, home nursing, special dwellings, alarm systems, aids/appliances and meals on wheels etc) are allocated on the basis of an individual assessment of need[2]. The most common criterion for allocation is the (in)ability to perform domestic and personal care tasks; the more incapacitated, the more help is allocated (Boll Hansen and Platz, 1995b). Home nursing requires a referral from a GP or hospital, while allocation of all other municipal services are dependent on an assessment of need by a supervising nurse or social worker. In principle, all referrals are handled by each municipality's central Committee on Social Welfare and Health. However, as a result of municipal reorganisations (see below), the allocation of services has in many places been decentralised. Now the supervising nurse or social worker at district level is likely to be able to allocate whatever domiciliary services they deem necessary, and will make recommendations to the municipality's central committee about the allocation of nursing home places, adapted housing and technical aids (Eigil Boll Hansen, personal communications).

From institutional to domiciliary care and changes in the organisation of community care

This section first describes the policy of de-institutionalisation and the substitution of community for institutional services within municipalities. It then discusses changes in both community care and nursing home based services which have been introduced to support this substitution.

Substitution between services provided by municipalities

The aims of the 'in own home for as long as possible' policy were to promote specialised housing over institutional care, and to separate care and nursing services from issues of accommodation, so as to give older people the same services irrespective of whether they live at home or in institutions. This idea originated in an experimental project in the early 1980s (Wagner, 1989) and was enacted in the 1988 Housing for the Elderly Act. This halted investment and building in nursing homes and other accommodation with integral nursing care and laid down provision for the building of special dwellings for older people (Daatland, 1997).

The implementation of this policy has meant that municipalities have closed down nursing home places and either converted these into special dwellings or built new housing. To accommodate the increased demand on domiciliary services, municipalities have also developed their home care services, including extending service provision beyond daytime hours, providing access to emergency help (see Figure 6.1), establishing more day centres and opening nursing homes for day care.

Figure 6.1: 24-hour home care services or round-the-clock schemes

Care is provided to older people in their homes beyond traditional daytime hours. 24-hour services may include home nursing or home help or both. The extension of services may include evenings and/or nights. The schemes differ from one municipality to another, but consist in principle of two elements: an emergency scheme which can be called 24 hours a day; and a visiting service at agreed times of the day or night (Plovsing, 1992). Round-the-clock services were introduced in individual municipalities as far back as the late 1970s. Today they are provided in 97% of municipalities (Felbo and Søland, 1996).

How comprehensive has this substitution between services been? Has inadequate substitution of community-based services resulted in unmet needs? There have been three major concerns concerning gaps in provision: whether, with the reduction in nursing home places, there is enough accommodation suitable for frail older people; whether the type and amount of home care services are adequate; and finally whether the policy of 'in own home for as long as possible' has led to increased problems of loneliness among older people or created new needs for psychological and emotional care (Plovsing, 1992). The extent to which these concerns are warranted is probably the most thoroughly investigated aspect of Danish policy for older people.

Research carried out in the early 1990s following the implementation of the Housing for the Elderly Act, of the housing policies of 246 of the 275 municipalities indicated that there was a shortfall in provision for older people who needed special housing or nursing home places. Approximately 12,000 older people were on waiting lists for special dwellings, indicating that full substitution was some way off (Platz, 1992a; 1992b; Platz and Petersen, 1992). However, recent surveys indicate that although there has been a tightening of criteria for the allocation of nursing home places, this shortfall has become less of a problem. From 1991 to 1995, the overall provision of accommodation suitable for frail older people (nursing homes and adapted dwellings) fell by 0.2% relative to the number of older people. However, when municipalities' plans for new accommodation are taken into account, coverage will be the same by 1997 as it was in 1991 (Boll Hansen and Platz, 1995a). Furthermore, overall there has been no increase in the number of physically frail older people living in their own homes since the passing of the Act, approximately 20% in both 1988 and 1994. Nor has there been a rise in the proportion of older people living in ordinary or special dwellings who think they have bad health (Boll Hansen and Platz, 1995b; 1996).

As regards the type and amount of home care services, the concern has been whether domiciliary care services have been able to keep pace with the increasing number of older people who need these following the ending of investment in nursing homes. However, by 1998 almost all municipalities had 24-hour home care services. Moreover, the overriding conclusion from evaluation studies is that neither home nursing nor home help services have become more difficult to obtain. On the contrary, in 1994 relatively more older people received home nursing compared with 1988; there has also been an increase in the proportion of older people living alone who receive home help (Boll Hansen and Platz, 1995a; 1995b; Daatland, 1997). However, there has been a drastic reduction in the number of hours of home help allocated to each person and a consequent prioritisation of help with personal care at the expense of domestic help (Ministry of Social Affairs, 1991; Ministry of Trade and Industry et al, 1995; Boll Hansen and Platz, 1995a), particularly help with cleaning, cooking and shopping (Boll Hansen and Platz, 1995b). A contributing factor has been the reorganisation of home helps into semi-autonomous working groups which has been carried out with (slightly) hidden cutbacks (Lewinter, in press; 1997a; 1997b). Moreover, domestic help is now given less on a routine basis and more in response to individual needs. These changes indicate a targeting of resources towards older people with greater care needs.

As a result, there is considerably greater dissatisfaction among users, with as many as 40% claiming they receive insufficient help with practical tasks (Boll Hansen and Platz, 1995b). A particular concern is that help with cleaning is not received as agreed (Kock-Nielsen and Nørregård, 1992). Older people also express dissatisfaction about the lack of continuity in home helps (Odense Kommune, 1995; Tilia, 1995; Udviklingskontoret, 1994). In contrast, all the indications are that users feel they receive enough help with personal care and home nursing (Boll Hansen and Platz, 1995b).

The core of domiciliary care services are home nursing and home help which are free of charge. However, some municipalities have responded to continuing increased demands for domestic home help by introducing extra services for which users must pay. These include cleaning and laundry services, meals on wheels, the home supply of frozen food or access to a nursing home canteen (Boll Hansen and Platz, 1995a). These services are sometimes offered as supplements to other services; sometimes they replace services which home helps no longer provide.

Concerns that the policy of 'in own home for as long as possible', and the reduction in nursing home places in particular, may have led to increased problems of insecurity and loneliness have arisen for two reasons. First, the criteria used to allocate staffed dwellings and nursing home places take more account of an older person's physical health than their mental well-being and social networks (Boll Hansen and Platz, 1996); second, reductions in the amount of time for which home helps visit may have reduced for many older people their only source of social contact, particularly in urban areas (Leeson, 1997). However, it has recently been shown that feelings of insecurity or loneliness are independent of the form of accommodation; there are as many older people in nursing homes as in other forms of accommodation who feel insecure, afraid or lonely. Overall, the proportion of older people feeling lonely was lower in 1994 than ever before (Boll Hansen and Platz, 1995b; 1996).

Hence, although there was some reason for concern in the early stages of the substitution process, more recent evidence indicates that by the mid-1990s it has been accomplished largely without leaving major gaps in provision, apart from the reduction of domestic services for older people in their own homes.

Denmark followed a pattern of substitution, where reductions in institutional care are (more or less) substituted by expansion in community services. (Daatland, 1997, p 166 – English summary)

Towards an integrated system for the delivery of community care

Nursing homes, home help and home nursing are all the responsibility of municipalities. Traditionally, they were administered in separate organisational structures within the municipality, each with its own leader, budget and aims (Wagner, 1995). However, the fact that these separate services were all funded and organised at the same level of local government has facilitated substantial integration in the organisation of services in the wake of the de-institutionalisation policy.

This integration process has consisted of a series of separate but interrelated stages (Larsen, 1993; Danish Nurses' Organisation, 1989; 1991). These are described greater detail in Figure 6.2.

Figure 6.2: Stages in the process of integrating community care services

Functional, multi-disciplinary teams

All groups of personnel involved in home care for older people have been brought under the same administrative unit; at the same time the quality of professional teamwork improved as professionals were better educated (see below).

Decentralisation

The division of geographical areas into smaller self-governing districts, each with a team consisting of home nurses, home helps, occupational therapists etc led by a nurse. These teams are responsible for the everyday nursing service and other care services available to clients in the areas.

Joint operation scheme

The same professionals care for older people in nursing homes and in their own homes. 'Fully integrated' means that *all* staff groups (nurses, aides, home helps and occupational therapists etc) work across care settings 24 hours (day, evening and night). 'Moderated' schemes include schemes in which only one group of professionals works across domiciliary and nursing home boundaries (eg, nurses), or schemes in which staff work as integrated teams for only part of the 24-hour period, typically evenings and nights. In effect, the schemes mean abolishing the boundaries between institutions and home care; in principle, the personnel are expected to cover both forms in a district. This type of integration was piloted in around 20 municipalities during the 1980s (Danish Nurses' Organisation, 1991) and was formalised in 1989 through a re-negotiation of the collective agreement between the Danish Nurses' Organisation and the National Association of Municipalities (Larsen, 1993). Three years after joint operation was formalised, 181 municipalities had their home care and nursing home staff merged to let them serve all older people (Larsen, 1993, p 23). By 1995, 75% of municipalities had implemented joint operation schemes (Eigil Boll Hansen, personal communication).

New educational structure

Joint operation schemes have been supported by the introduction of a new, more streamlined educational system in 1993 which means that personnel serving older people in 'old' nursing homes and in ordinary housing stock now receive the same training. The new structure also increased the level of training received by helping professionals. For example, employment requirements for home helps increased from a seven-week course to a full year.

From nursing home to health centre

In some places the nursing home has changed role to a health centre. This has more elements to it. With the 1988 Housing for the Elderly Act, older people moving to nursing homes could keep their family doctor rather than change to the GP attached to the nursing hom e. In 1993 new legislation (lov nr 112 af 22.12.93) was introduced so that, rather than contributing their full pension to their upkeep in a nursing home, which is a total service package, residents receive their pensions directly and are expected to pay for food, hairdressing, personal purchases, medicine etc (Wagner, 1994). In some places it also means that rooms have been converted into private flats and centres for social activities, physio- and occupational therapy, kitchen and laundry (Danish Nurses' Organisation, 1991). This new concept has been adopted, partly or totally, by approximately 75% of the municipalities in Denmark (Wagner, 1997). These centres often form the physical base for staff of joint operation schemes. A precondition for the establishment of joint operation schemes is a 24-hour home care service. The organisation of joint operation schemes often involves dividing a municipality into a number of self-governing areas with functional teams, eg, around a nursing home.

These integration measures started as pilot projects in individual municipalities during the 1980s but have been adopted on a wider basis in line with the de-institutionalisation policy. By the mid-1990s, the integration of the home help and nursing services in a decentralised structure had been adopted most widely; joint operation schemes and the new nursing home concept had been adopted in at least three quarters of municipalities.

A fully integrated service would look something like this. The municipality has de-centralised day-to-day responsibility for community services to an autonomous district, based around a nursing home. The nursing home has been converted into a health centre which provides a physical base for staff. The notion of separating care from housing has been extended to residents in nursing homes. Staff, organised in multi-disciplinary teams of both home helps and nurses, care both for residents in adapted flats linked to the health centre and people in the surrounding area who live in their own homes or in purpose built municipal accommodation. People living in their own homes as well as those living in the former nursing home have access to help in the evenings and during the night; in emergencies they can call the '24-hour central office' to request help from home helps, home nurses and so on, free of charge.

An important factor for the success of the integration process has been a political willingness to pilot new ideas; municipalities which have wished to support research projects have received funding from the Ministry of Social Affairs for both the project and its evaluation. The earliest initiative to implement the full package, which is also the project from which many of the ideas originate, was in a small municipality (Skævinge) in 1984. The project involved both the establishment of 24-hour services for the whole community and the conversion of a former nursing home into a health centre with sheltered flats, guest flats and a day centre open to all citizens. Evaluations of this initiative (Wagner, 1989; 1992; 1994; 1995; 1997), of individual pilots in 24 hours services (Boll Hansen and Werborg, 1984a; 1984b; 1985), and of joint operation schemes (Boll Hansen et al, 1991), have to a large extent focused on resource implications, utilisation of services and professional attitudes. They have also confirmed the benefits for older people, such as better coordinated care, continuity of care and increased choice and autonomy for older people both outside and within institutionalised care.

Development of 24-hour domiciliary services, together with the possibility of moving to adapted housing specifically suited to the needs of frail older people, clearly contribute to increased choice for older people, particularly the choice to remain at home, which is what most people prefer (Wagner, 1995; 1997). Evaluations of some of the earliest 24-hour services indicate that the schemes also increased older people's sense of security (Boll Hansen and Werborg, 1984b; 1985).

If an older person needs to go into a nursing home, the joint operation scheme has the potential to ease the move, as the same staff continue to care for them[3]. This increases continuity of care for the older people, which may be a central precondition for agreeing to go into a nursing home even if only for a short stay (Wagner, 1994).

The changes in the roles of nursing homes are on the whole intended to create parity between older people in nursing homes and those living independently. Thus, the person maintains the same conditions as they had when living in a non-institutional setting in terms of individualised care, self-determination and autonomy. For example, rather than having to contribute their full pension in return for a uniform package of care, nursing home residents today receive their pensions directly and pay only for the services they want or need individually, thus creating a more individualised package of care (Rold Andersen, 1993) and retaining social and economic autonomy (Wagner, 1997).

Overall, this substitution policy has led to increased integration and coordination of community-based care within municipalities.

Improving the transition across the interface between hospital and community-based care

Another interface is that between community care and hospital care, which is funded and operated separately by the counties. Responsibilities for hospital care and for care once patients leave hospital are divided between county and municipality levels of local government. This has led to mutual claims of cost shunting; counties claim that municipalities try to keep the older people in hospital longer than necessary, while municipalities claim that hospitals discharge patients too soon.

The main problems include admission of older people to hospitals for inappropriate 'social' reasons: such as pressure from families, to give the GP or home help some respite, or because deputising GPs do not know the individuals; 'bed-blocking' as a result of the reduction in the number of nursing home places and lack of other appropriate arrangements for frail older people in the municipalities; and insufficient rehabilitation in both hospitals and municipalities (Alban et al, 1988; Felbo and Søland, 1996; Association of County Councils and National Association of Municipalities, 1991).

New models of cooperation

These problems are beginning to be addressed (Sejr et al, 1995; Boll Hansen et al, 1997; Felbo and Søland, 1996) and many examples of good practice to improve the overall coherence and continuity of care for older people have been identified – see Figure 6.3.

Figure 6.3: Initiatives to improve coordination for older people who need hospital care

Initiatives to reduce number of hospital and nursing home admissions

- Increased emphasis on *outreach*: early initiative piloted in individual municipalities includes home visits by a geriatric team (Hansen, 1993) and outreach nurses for people over 78 years old who do not receive home care. From Summer 1996 all municipalities are obliged to offer two annual home visits for check-up to those over 80-years-old as part of their home care services.

- Individual municipalities have piloted schemes which involve *rehabilitation and/or relief stays in elderly centres* for older people who need rehabilitation and training in connection with a spell of ill-health or who need a short stay in an institution. One municipality has established the possibility for self-referral to an acute care department in a nursing home and another has established an option for GPs and district nurses to refer older people to an acute stay in a residential centre or establish round-the-clock observation in the home. These initiatives have been shown to represent important alternatives to hospital and/or nursing home admissions in spells of acute illness, as supplements to the municipality's 24-hour home care service (Boll Hansen et al, 1997).

Initiatives to improve continuity between hospitals and municipality services

- **Payment:** in many areas the municipalities now have to pay the counties for each day an older person stays in hospital after medical treatment is over.

- **A coordination nurse** employed in the home help organisation in the municipality visits the hospital daily in order to coordinate care between hospital and municipality. This initiative has been shown to reduce older people's use of institutions and improve their sense of security (Hendriksen and Strømgård, 1989; Hendriksen et al, 1989). Similar results have been found where the district nurse and the GP each pay one home visit to older people shortly after discharge (Hansen et al, 1994).

- **'Good coordination practice'** in which procedures around hospital admissions and discharge are agreed between the hospital and municipalities in the catchment area of the hospital (Boll Hansen et al, 1997).

Most of these initiatives have been piloted only in individual areas and are far from universal, and only a few of the schemes have been systematically evaluated. In particular, information is missing about older people's experience of these schemes (Sejr et al, 1995; Boll Hansen et al, 1997).

Interface between municipal and non-public services

As already noted, in Denmark most care-giving functions are considered a public responsibility. Neither voluntary organisations or the private sector plays any significant role (Plovsing, 1992). Private sector involvement has been limited to not-for-profit, non-religious humanitarian organisations involved in running institutions, but with funding responsibilities still lying firmly within the public domain. Voluntary organisations have mainly social functions, such as organising 'visiting friends' or 'telephone chains' for lonely older people, and giving telephone advice. Informal carers play a somewhat bigger role in care-giving for older people, although with a clear division of labour from the municipal home help. Informal carers often help with administrative tasks such as personal finance and contact with municipal services, and with domestic tasks such as shopping and laundry. Less common is help with personal care, which is the domain of the home help (Lewinter, 1997c; in preparation; Boll Hansen and Platz, 1995b)[4].

However, in recent years there have been two unprecedented developments, both of which are intended to break the monopoly of municipalities in the provision of services for older people. This is part of a broader trend to increase the welfare mix and develop quasi-markets in social care, in order to manage an anticipated increase in demand arising from demographic changes in the numbers and changes in the characteristics of the population of older people within the constraints of public spending limits. One development involves new models of cooperation between municipal professionals and voluntary organisations in local services for older people. This is part of a larger programme supported by the Ministry of Social Affairs (Swane, 1994). Initiatives include trained volunteers who offer support to families caring for people with dementia, support older people in the first days at home after discharge from hospitals, or provide counselling (Leeson, 1997).

This programme seems to have influenced attitudes of both national and local policy makers to the involvement of voluntary organisations (Swane, 1994), but has not extended to doing work traditionally carried out by professionals employed by municipalities (Anker and Kock-Nielsen, 1995; Rasmussen, 1997). For example, with respect to the support of the relatives of older people with dementia (one of the most common types of initiative), involvement has been largely limited to providing a couple of hours volunteer respite help in the evenings or weekends so that family members can go shopping or attend family events (Elisabeth Toft Rasmussen, personal communications). The main reason for this is an overall consensus among both voluntary workers and public employees that tasks such as home help are professional activities and should be paid as such (Rasmussen, 1997).

A second, and much more controversial initiative in recent years is the 'privatisation' which has taken place in relation to home care services. This 'privatisation' includes both the introduction of extra home help services (over and above the statutory minimum) for which there is a co-payment by the user (Rønnow, 1996), the contracting out to private companies of the standard home care services, and, in one case, the leasing-out of municipal nursing homes (*Jyllands-Posten*, 1997; *Fyns Stiftidende*, 1997a; 1997b). In all instances, financing and overall responsibility remain in the public sector, while greater competition is encouraged in the provision of services. In most cases users can choose between public and private service providers.

However, the contracting-out movement has not progressed as far as anticipated. Only a handful of municipalities have contracted out services for elderly people to private companies and most are restricted to practical home help services. The number of municipalities offering extra services for additional co-payments is also very limited and the number of municipalities who offer traditional home help services only as an extra service for a fee is negligible (Rønnow, 1996; Boll Hansen and Platz, 1995a). One reason is concern among municipal employees and their unions about changes in their terms and conditions of work (Ministry of Interior/Home Affairs, 1997). A second reason is the threat to the autonomy and integration of self-managed district teams and joint operation practices, particularly the reduction in professional discretion when detailed service specifications are developed as part of the contracting out process.

A further influence is the attitudes of users. A recent study in three municipalities showed that although there may be a tentative acceptance of co-payments for services, there is distinct resistance to the idea that profit should be made from welfare services, particularly in relation to vulnerable older people (Rønnow, 1996). Finally there are threats to the political interests of municipal councils, as they lose control of the day-to-day running of the services and, with that, the possibility of intervention in individual cases for political reasons (for example, boosting popularity in the period up to local election).

Nevertheless, these are potentially significant developments. The most pressing concerns are about the potential impact on the integration of community-based services which has been achieved within municipalities over the last decades. Professional concerns focus on the threat to self-managed integrated teams, while another important issue concerns the potential impact on individualised, coordinated care and continuity of care schemes (Lis Wagner, personal communication). There are anxieties over the increasing standardisation of services which results from tight service specifications, in contrast to the individualised care which is possible when some degree of discretion is left to professionals. It is not clear whether professionals in privatised services will be able to detect needs for further help. A particular concern is the threat to outreach and preventive work for very frail older people who are not able to seek help of their own; how will they fare without a structured outreach system within public sector services?

Furthermore, the privatisation of just the home help service jeopardises coordination, because it breaks up integrated teams into a group caring for older people who only need practical help and one for those who need domestic, personal and nursing care (Rønnow, 1996). A further concern is the threat to continuity in the joint operation schemes: if services such as personal care or nursing are contracted out, will it be possible for the same helper to follow an older person if and when they go into a nursing home, which is currently possible if the older person moves to a nursing home within the catchment area of the scheme?

These potential implications have not been explored in any detail; evaluations so far have focused on user satisfaction. Indications are that there is a high degree of satisfaction with the services provided by the private companies. However, it is important to note that great care has been taken in the pilot contracting-out schemes to ensure that quality of care is maintained; this includes detailed service specifications and quality indicators, user satisfaction targets of 80%, extensive monitoring arrangements such as control visits and complaints monitoring, and firm sanctions which include the termination of contracts if quality criteria are not satisfied (Ministry of Interior/Home Affairs, 1997). It is not clear whether these high standards will be maintained if schemes extend beyond the demonstration project stage.

Conclusions

What has been the overall impact of these changes on the quality of life, choice and autonomy of older people, on their access to services and social inclusion?

The substitution process which followed the de-institutionalisation policy has increased the diversity of services which has in turn increased choice for older people. The major components of this have been the emphasis on housing as an integral part of community care policies and the extension of home care to a round-the-clock rather than a daytime only service. Thus 20 years ago, if more than domestic and personal care services were needed, older people would be offered a place in a nursing home. Today, most municipalities provide housing specifically adapted for older people and 24-hour home care services. There is therefore an alternative to going into a nursing home for even very disabled, frail or confused older people.

The changes in the organisation of municipalities' services have meant that the enlarged range of services are also more integrated, with greater emphasis on coordination and continuity of care. In addition, the changing concept of nursing homes, which developed as part of these reorganisations, has meant that to a large degree older people maintain their social and economic independence when entering a nursing home. These achievements were inspired by the visionary ideas which emerged from the work of the Elder Commission in the early 1980s and have been facilitated by a political openness to innovation and financial support for pilot projects to test ideas prior to their adoption on a wider basis.

These are major improvements in terms of choice and self-determination and autonomy. They have been paralleled and enhanced with two other recent formal initiatives. First, in response to widespread criticism of the amount and quality of home help given to older people, there has been a strengthening of the right to complain. From 1996 municipal councils are required explicitly to define the service package available locally, develop service specifications and set up local boards to hear complaints (Boll Hansen, 1997). A second development has been to formalise the political representation of older people's interests. From January 1997 municipalities have been obliged to establish locally elected 'elderly councils', whose remit is to advise the council on its elder policy and which must be consulted over any significant service changes (Jespersen, 1997). The rights to information and redress extend to most frail older people, while the 'elderly councils' are likely to involve only the younger, more resourceful and active part of the older population.

These positive outcomes have been achieved without altering fundamental entitlements. Thus home care services have expanded in scope without changes in conditions of access, apart from home help services where there has been a prioritisation of help with personal care over help with domestic cleaning, cooking and shopping. Ease of access and the amount of help given with home nursing and personal care has remained unchanged. In respect of domestic home help services, it has not become more difficult to obtain services – in fact, a growing number of older people receive it – but the service is spread more thinly.

This does not mean that there are no negative outcomes. Greater coordination and integration in service provision within municipalities could, if great care is not taken, lead to more problems in coordinating services between municipal services and county level hospitals (Alban et al, 1988; Felbo and Søland, 1996). Some of the initiatives to reduce boundary problems have been adopted more or less universally, such as payments by municipalities to counties for older people who remain in hospital after they are ready for discharge. Other initiatives, such as increased emphasis on outreach work from municipal home care services, have been formalised in national legislation or regulations. However, many examples of good practice, including the provision of intermediate forms of care, remain isolated initiatives.

This raises the issue of variations in service provision locally. Improvements in the coordination of care between hospital and community services are in some areas still patchy. To what extent are the improvements in municipal community care services universal throughout the country? As a result of the principle of 'self-governing local councils' there are variations across municipalities in the particular service packages available locally. However, this is not an issue of great concern in Denmark. One factor is that it can be difficult to see exactly what the differences are; the issue is therefore not as salient as in other more visible areas such as hospital waiting lists. Another factor is that variation is less a question of the type of services that are available locally, but rather whether the services available suit local circumstances. Recent evidence shows that differences between municipalities reflect the fact that different services have developed to meet local needs (Boll Hansen and Platz, 1995a; 1995b). The principle of 'self-governing local councils' seems to have a real content. Most important, however, may be the fact that there are no significant differences between municipalities in either access to services or the charges which are made for them.

The final concern is the potential impact of municipal initiatives to manage increased demand in the face of limited resources – that is, the trends in some municipalities to introduce extra services for which older people have to pay, to compensate for the reduction in domestic home help services, and the contracting out of part of their community care services to private companies. These developments pose a threat to the individualised, coordinated care which has been achieved through the integrated community care services. Both initiatives also harbour the potential for social exclusion. To the extent that extra services substitute for tasks no longer provided by home helps, these represent an erosion of entitlement to universally free welfare benefits, and thus a favouring of older people who can afford to pay at the expense of the less affluent. Furthermore, while competition to public sector service monopolies may increase choice, it may well be only the affluent older people who are able to shop around for quality services, while the less resourceful and less well off end up with poorer services.

The future challenge in Denmark is how these issues will be tackled if and when schemes like these are implemented on a wider scale.

Notes

[1] For example, expenditure administered by local government constitutes just 30% of total production (GDP), and just over half (52%) of total public expenditure; and local government tax revenue amounts to 31% of total public tax revenue (National Association of Municipalities, 1997).

[2] When allocating home help services, the municipality will normally take into account the practical help contributed by a spouse, but if the older person lives alone, possible help from other family members is not taken into account (Boll Hansen, 1997).

[3] This is the intention in the municipalities which have implemented joint operation schemes. However, practical circumstances, particularly in larger municipalities, may mean that continuity of care cannot be achieved in practice, for example, because of a shortage of nursing home places within a district. Therefore there may be a trade-off between continuity of care and immediate access to a place in a nursing home within the catchment area of the scheme (Eigil Boll Hansen, personal communication).

[4] While there have been numerous studies of formal care-giving, family care-giving has not been an important topic of study in Denmark. The prevalent belief, based primarily on interviews with older people themselves, has been that, due to the fact that in most cases both sons and daughters will have full-time jobs, the family (except spouses) played a limited role in care-giving for older people, their input being limited to social and psychological support and help to obtain public services (Platz and Petersen, 1992). However, recent interview surveys with relatives of older people (Lewinter, in preparation; 1997c; Boll Hansen and

Platz, 1995b) challenge that notion, in that the informal carer's role is shown to extend to a series of domestic tasks. Up to 70% of older people receive some form of help from relatives – who are most often children but who may also be other family members as well as neighbours and friends. About 50% receive help on a weekly basis. The specific division of labour found between informal carers and the municipal home help may be indicative of the reduction in home help hours allocated to individual older people, although it is not possible to say from existing data.

SEVEN

Acute and continuing care for older people in Australia: contesting new balances of care[1]

Michael Fine

Introduction

Developments in Australia in the last decades of the 20th century have seen aged care move from the margins of policy to the centre stage of political contest. It will be argued that aged care has been undergoing a far-reaching transformation. These changes reflect an ongoing contest by different groups and interests, the outcomes shaped by the pre-existing institutional infrastructure as much as by perceived demographic or economic imperatives.

The chapter focuses on developments associated with the emergence of community care and the attempts to incorporate this care into the broader health system. It traces the establishment of community care in Australia as a distinctive form of service provision from the 1960s onwards and subsequently examines its attempted incorporation into the broader system of health and extended care in the 1990s. While there is evidence of the successful establishment of links between community care, residential care and hospital-based services, considerable difficulties still remain.

Policy making in a federation

To understand developments in the Australian system of health and welfare, it is important to grasp two fundamental principles. The first concerns the Australian Constitution which sets out the division of responsibility between the Commonwealth (Australian or Federal) government and the

State and Territory governments. Under the 1901 constitution, healthcare is a responsibility of State governments. State governments are responsible for the licensing of all medical and paramedical practitioners and for the licensing and registration of all health facilities. In addition, State governments are responsible for the direct provision of health services through their Departments of Health. These include government owned public hospitals and community health services and a wide range of hospitals and services operated by non-government voluntary bodies (Grant and Lapsley, 1993).

However, the Commonwealth government has gradually assumed an increasingly important role in the financing, organisation and provision of care. In the postwar period, the Commonwealth government assumed responsibility for the regulation and subsidy of private health insurance and shortly afterwards the subsidy of nursing home care. Later governments have expanded this contribution significantly, with the direct funding of a range of community services and, most importantly, the introduction of first Medibank (1975) and later Medicare (1983), which provide free or nearly free access to healthcare for all Australians. Through its control of taxation revenue in Australia, the Commonwealth has also been in a position to exert a powerful influence over all aspects of healthcare financing and hence nearly all aspects of healthcare provision (Grant and Lapsley, 1993; Palmer and Short, 1994).

The second important feature of the Australian health and community care system is the interplay between public, voluntary and private concerns. Unlike many European countries, the Australian system has operated as a mixed market of public, voluntary and private concerns throughout this century, largely continuing a pattern that has its origins in the previous century (Sax, 1984; Palmer and Short, 1994). As Table 7.1 suggests, it would be incorrect to posit some sort of universal secular trend towards increased private responsibility for expenditure. Reflecting the dynamic between Commonwealth and State governments, an important feature of the table is the increase in the proportion of finance directly attributable to the Commonwealth government and the modest decline in the proportion of expenditure from State government sources.

Table 7.1: Changes in the proportion of public and private spending on healthcare (total health expenditure, 1982/83 to 1992/93)

Year	Commonwealth government	State and local government	Private	Total amount Aust$m
		%		
1982/83	38.4	26.9	34.7	13,239
1987/88	44.1	26.0	29.9	23,328
1992/93	44.3	23.5	32.2	34,338

Source: AIHW (1994a, p 8)

A slightly different indicator, the proportion of occupied bed days in acute hospitals (Table 7.2) shows a slight shift away from the use of public hospitals (ie, government and non-profit hospitals associated with State Departments of Health) and a corresponding increase in the use of private hospitals, over the same period.

Table 7.2: Hospital utilisation: occupied bed days in acute hospitals (1982/83 to 1991/92, all age groups)

Year	All public hospitals	Private hospitals
1982/83	17,940,990	4,839,187
1987/88	16,979,074	4,531,000
1991/92	15,637,664	5,042,230
	%	%
Average annual growth rate 1982/83 to 1991/92	-1.5	+0.5

Source: AIHW (1994b, p 6)

Unfortunately, published national statistics do not readily capture the full complexity of patterns of provision in Australian healthcare nor the changes to these in recent years (Fine, 1995c). For example, national figures on the proportion of public hospitals in each State operated by religious orders and non-profit trusts are not separated from those of public hospitals. Neither do statistics adequately convey a sense of the operational characteristics of the Australian healthcare system, in which the provision of healthcare is the direct product of the system of professional medical registration boards and the control exercised by the medical profession through the promotion of private practice and a fee-for-service system of payments for medical care (Palmer and Short, 1994). Within this pluralistic, heterogeneous system, the dynamics of policy development are continually subjected to the interplay of the different interests involved – particularly, in this instance, between the different types of providers. It has been necessary to search for ways and mechanisms which allow individuals to move with relative ease between public, voluntary and private-for-profit services.

Community care and the growth of the aged care industry

The origins of the current systems of both residential care and community support can be traced back to the Menzies Liberal/Country Party government which sought to honour a promise that it would "provide an effective bulwark against the socialisation of medicine" (Kewley, 1973, p 507, cited in Sax, 1984, p 60). To achieve this the Commonwealth government instituted the 1952 Hospital Benefits Act and a national system of voluntary health insurance in 1953. These moves effectively excluded many aged and disabled people from the hospitals on which they had relied for long-term care. In what has subsequently proved to be the birth of the Australian aged care industry (a term used by both government and organisations of nursing home proprietors), a series of somewhat ad hoc facilities emerged to provide for those who could not be cared for elsewhere. These were largely disused properties converted into 'rest homes' and 'convalescent homes' by private operators seeking to make a profit, charitable homes established in properties owned and controlled by the churches, and older State government facilities, including previous benevolent asylums and hospitals for infectious diseases. At the time, only a few of these were eligible to receive funding from Commonwealth hospital benefits. This led to the introduction of Commonwealth funded 'nursing home benefits' in 1963 (Sax, 1984) which effectively incorporated a large number of private facilities into the Commonwealth government system. At the same time the use of payments made directly to the nursing home proprietors confirmed a trend for the Commonwealth government to circumvent constitutional constraints on its direct provision of services.

The results of this open-ended commitment by the Commonwealth to subsidise non-government nursing homes were that the number of nursing home beds grew at a far greater rate than that of the aged population in general (Saunders and Fine, 1992). The number of private, profit-making ventures grew particularly vigorously, as entrepreneurs realised the opportunity provided by a government guaranteed income.

Table 7.3: Total number of nursing home beds in Australia (1963-94)

Year	1963	1968	1972	1978	1983	1988	1990	1994
All nursing homes	25,535	37,883	53,416	58,482	72,599	72,116	72,615	74,257
Combined voluntary and private homes	16,130	26,051	38,224	44,864	57,530	58,951	59,649	62,079
Private homes	n/a	n/a	28,799	28,717	34,384	34,900	34,699	35,198
State government homes	9,405	11,832	10,833	13,615	18,069	13,165	12,966	12,178

Source: Senate Select Committee (1984); DHHCS (1991); AIHW (1995)

Despite a series of reforms commenced in the early 1970s, the number of nursing home beds continued to grow until, by the early 1980s, Australia was said to have the greatest number of nursing home beds per head of the aged population in the world (Saunders and Fine, 1992; DCS, 1986). The level of expenditure required to maintain this stock of beds left little scope for alternative forms of support, such as those provided by community care services. The poor standards of care found in many nursing homes were attributed by many observers to problems in the payment of nursing home benefits and the reluctance of the Commonwealth government to take action (Senate Select Committee, 1984; Parker, 1987). Part of this reluctance arose from the fact that the State governments continued to be responsible under the Australian Constitution for licensing nursing homes, not the Commonwealth government which provided the funding.

Community care services, like nursing homes, also developed under a model of direct Commonwealth government finance and non-government provision, with the important difference that services were largely provided by locally-based, non-profit, voluntary organisations. For-profit service providers were not beneficiaries of government funds. The current system can be traced back to the 1957 Home Nursing Subsidy Scheme, under which the Commonwealth government paid the salary costs of all home nurses employed up to that date, and half the salary of all new home nurses employed afterwards. Other sources of funds for these services were grants from the State governments, and fees paid by patients (McLeay, 1982, p 12). This model was elaborated in later developments, which shared the costs of financing services such as home care and paramedical care between the Commonwealth and State governments. The 1970 Delivered Meals Subsidy Act, in contrast, involved a direct payment from the Commonwealth government to services operated by voluntary organisations and local government bodies.

If these schemes were intended to foster the development of community care on a large scale, they proved inadequate in practice. The system of public finance which operated until the early 1980s encouraged the provision of nursing home places, particularly in the for-profit sector, but restricted the growth of services to people who remained in their own home (Fine and Stevens, 1998). Nursing homes were funded directly by the Commonwealth on the basis of daily fees for each resident, which provided an incentive to maximise usage rates. In contrast, the mechanisms for public funding of community support services generally involved a complex, centralised and restrictive system, in which a limited number of block grants were awarded by the Commonwealth government on an annual basis to specific organisations (Fine et al, 1991). The result was a substantial imbalance towards nursing homes and away from community care. Even more important, aged care represented a system in which the Commonwealth government financed and was held responsible for the system of services, but did not exert effective control over the most significant elements of the system – the admission of patients to nursing homes or the distribution or level of provision of nursing home facilities.

To overcome these problems, a number of important reforms were introduced by the new Labour government into the long-term care system for older people in the mid-1980s. These included the introduction of restrictions on the provision and use of nursing homes, tighter entry criteria and standardised assessment procedures, the introduction of a form of casemix funding which linked payments received by nursing home proprietors to the dependency levels of residents and the development of specialised multi-disciplinary Aged Care Assessment Teams (ACATs). Perhaps most importantly, a new, revitalised approach was taken to the provision of community care with the introduction of the Home and Community Care Program (HACC). This programme, designed to provide an expanded range of services to people who require support to remain living independently in their own homes, involved a system of block payments to locally-based non-profit agencies, the cost of which was shared by the Commonwealth and State governments (DHHCS, 1991).

These measures saw a marked shift in Australian policy for aged care towards community support, with greater emphasis on assessment and targeting as a means of ensuring that individuals receive appropriate services while tight budgetary constraints were maintained. As a result of these changes, a gradual shift in expenditure in favour of community care took place. In the early 1980s, 11 dollars was spent on nursing homes and hostels for every 1 dollar spent on community care (McLeay, 1982, p 123). By 1991 this ratio had changed to 4.7:1. According to projections made at the time, if these policies were maintained, this would become a ratio of approximately 3:1 by the year 2001 (DHHCS, 1991; Fine, 1995b).

Since 1996, much of the focus of policy has been to try to reduce the extent of the Commonwealth's financial commitment to aged care. Perhaps the most dramatic expression of this came in the proposal that all health and aged care matters should be made a State government responsibility. However, this proposal was ultimately rejected by all State governments, fearful of the cost implications of such an undertaking (AIHW, 1997). The State government's reluctance seemed vindicated when moves in 1997 by the Commonwealth government to impose high entry fees on nursing home applicants and increase resident charges within nursing homes proved to be so enormously unpopular that their full implementation was reviewed and delayed until at least mid-1998.

Searching for the missing link: coordinating aged, acute and primary care

With the expansion and enhancement of community care services through the HACC programme, Australia could be said to have acquired all the elements of a comprehensive and complex health and extended care system. Yet accusations of cost-shifting between State and Commonwealth funded programmes and between private and public service providers are still rife, and evidence of serious imbalances and misallocations in the use of resources has continued to mount. Efforts to reduce these costs have threatened to shift costs on to other alternative services which, in effect, act as substitute provisions.

The fragmentation of health and community services has, in fact, been recognised as a problem for policy makers, service providers and consumers in Australia for many years (NHS, 1991; Fine, 1995a). As efforts to alter the balance of health and welfare services have run up against barriers created by the existing divisions between services and programmes, calls for change have become increasingly urgent. The apparent discontinuity between acute care provided in hospitals and ongoing care provided by community support and other extended care services has received particular attention in recent years. In submissions made to a recent official inquiry, for example, it was argued that developments such as the reduced length of stay in hospital, the trend towards early discharge and the increasing incidence of day surgery have placed considerable pressure on the community care system (Morris, 1994, pp 81-4). Similar claims were made to the inquiry by providers of residential care who, like their community care counterparts, argued that they have been compelled to provide what is in effect a form of post-acute care at the expense of long-term care recipients. Fears were also expressed that the widespread introduction of casemix funding in healthcare would increase pressures to shift the costs of care from hospital budgets to community and residential care services. Documentation of these problems has, however, been poor and inconsistent (Morris, 1994).

Nevertheless there have been a number of attempts to remedy the fragmentation of services and overcome the barriers to more coordinated, effective and efficient services. A range of innovative schemes are either currently being considered or have already been implemented, to try and optimise service use following discharge from hospital (Figure 7.1).

Figure 7.1: Approaches to Australian post-acute care

Type of approach	Practical example
• Discharge planning	In-hospital procedures
• Transfer payments	Casemix payments
	Purchase of service arrangements: eg Transition Care Projects (TCP), Medicare Incentive Packages (MIP)
• Organisational arrangements	Contracting out
	Cooperation with external agencies
	In-house provision
• Large-scale system redesign	Coordinated care trials

Discharge planning

Perhaps the most straightforward, widely implemented and well recognised of attempts to link hospital and other extended care provisions is that of discharge planning. The basic approach is entirely procedural, concerned with activities that need to be followed within hospitals prior to finalising the discharge of patients from the hospital ward. Best practice guidelines setting out both agreed principles for discharge planning and a guide for the development of post-discharge care policies are currently being prepared by the Commonwealth Department of Health and Family Services (DHFS, 1996) and have recently been used by the Commonwealth Department in an educational initiative, to provide the basis for a national approach. Nonetheless, departmental staff report that there are already a number of models being used, each of which has been developed to suit particular circumstances. Among these are the approach adopted by the Prince of Wales Hospital in Sydney, in which the hospital directly provides post-acute care services; that of the Royal Melbourne Hospital, in which an independent organisation which has close links with the hospital coordinates and purchases services from other providers; and the DAART approach, adopted in Brisbane, where a community service provides ongoing services for a number of hospitals.

A useful example of the general approach of discharge planning is provided in the report *Removing the boundaries: Hospital discharge practices and older people returning to the community* by the Council on the Ageing (Victoria) (COTA, 1994). Pointing to the increasing importance of ensuring continuity of care between hospital and home as the roles of the health services undergo rapid change, the report sets out eight principles of good discharge planning, which are summarised in Figure 7.2. As the report points out, implementation of most of these principles lies largely in the control of hospital personnel. Their effectiveness is also dependent on the voluntary cooperation of a wide range of non-hospital service providers. Not surprisingly, problems often arise when ongoing care is being planned, because services provided to those at home are currently organised and financed separately to those within hospitals.

Figure 7.2: Eight principles of good discharge planning

i.   Discharge planning must be an integral part of everyone's hospital care.

ii.   Older people, their families and carers should be involved as equal partners in the discharge process.

iii. Discharge planning should start on, or before, admission, and be based on appropriate systematic assessment questions.

iv. Information should be provided on discharge about the recovery path likely to be experienced on returning home.

v.   Information should be provided on discharge about services and programmes available in the community.

vi.   Discharge from hospital must be timely and linked to the responsiveness of post-acute care.

vii. Ongoing communication and coordination between hospitals and community-based services is essential for good discharge planning.

viii. Discharge planning must include support and information to carers.

Source: COTA (1994, pp 7-13, 45-88)

Transfer payments

A number of reports and reviews have suggested that the existing barriers to the use of community services by post-acute patients arise largely from the fragmented system of service funding (NHS, 1991). With reimbursements for hospital treatment ceasing at the point of discharge, referral to community services, especially those funded through the HACC programme, is sometimes suspected of amounting to no more than cost-shifting. Many reformers have therefore, not surprisingly, looked to the adoption of various prospective payment systems such as casemix payments or transition care arrangements.

Casemix payments

Casemix classifications were first developed in the USA in the 1970s and early 1980s to classify, measure and compare the health outputs of different health facilities (Tatchell, 1983). Because of their capacity to synthesise a range of factors associated with the cost of providing treatment through the use of Diagnosis Related Groups (DRGs), casemix classifications have since been widely adopted as the preferred payment mechanism for episodes of hospital care in the US. They are also used extensively for research purposes in Australia and have increasingly been adopted as the basis for reimbursing episodes of hospital care. An important element in the success of casemix measures is the fact that reimbursement is linked to the average cost of care for a case or episode of illness, thus allowing service providers flexibility at the same time as ensuring significant incentives for efficiency. Rather than focusing on the inputs (such as staff activity) or intermediate outputs (patient days, admissions and so on), as occurs when payments are fee-for-service or linked to specific service mixes, casemix measures focus attention on the outcomes of the process of treatment for individuals with the same diagnoses and conditions within comparable service settings (Tatchell, 1983; Eagar, 1996).

However, it may be less appropriate to extend hospital casemix payments to cover post-hospital care needs, because these needs are not predicted by the diagnosis but are more dependent on the individual's personal, social and economic circumstances. Hindle and Gillett (1993), for example, have suggested that because older people are more likely to suffer multiple conditions, their major diagnosis, even with allowance made for 'complicating conditions', is a poor predictor of their needs for ongoing care. Similarly, other non-disease attributes, such as the degree of functional disability, the availability of social supports and the suitability of housing, each of which is a significant determinant of the need for help among older people, are not taken into account. To date, in Australia the use of casemix payments has been largely a matter of discussion and experimentation, rather than practical implementation. Donnelly et al (1995), for example, developed a classification of episodes of care which explained up to 33.16% of the variation in costs when overheads and travel were taken into consideration. While not yet advocating the adoption of these measures as the preferred form of payment for community care episodes, there appears to be much support for further work on the issue. Work is also proceeding in other projects, including the development of sub and non-acute casemix classifications through the SNAP project (Eager, 1996) and through the work of the Royal District Nursing Service in Melbourne (Maddox, 1996). Magennis et al (1994), for example, argue that there are many benefits to be obtained from the introduction of sub-acute casemix classifications, including the prevention of cost-shifting from hospitals to community agencies.

Direct purchase of services

The direct purchase of community services by hospital-based staff represents an alternative form of prospective payment that has received attention in recent years. In Australia, this has taken two main forms: Transition Care Projects (TCP) and Medicare Incentive Packages (MIPs). While each of these schemes is well known in the field, few of the reviews and evaluations conducted have yet found their way into the refereed or international literature.

The Transition Care Program was introduced by the Commonwealth Government in 1993. Six Transition Care Projects were established, one in each State, in which an Aged Care Assessment Team (ACAT) was provided with extra staffing for the management of the project and with a pool of funds with which to buy assistance from community services, to assist with the transition of elderly people from hospital to home.

The specific aim of TCP was:

> ... **to reduce the number of inappropriate admissions to residential care by targeting additional funding to short-term, intensive care and support services for high dependency older people, particularly those discharged from hospital....** (TCP Discussion Paper and Guidelines, 1993, cited in New South Wales Aged Care Assessment Program, 1996, para 3.70)

In this way the aim and target group were both similar to, but quite distinct from those which might be expected in a programme for post-acute care.

The available reports give a mixed picture of the effectiveness of the programme. The evaluation of the New South Wales project, the only one which a control group was available, concluded that the TCP intervention successfully facilitated access to a range of community services for hospital patients being discharged back into community settings, although it did not have an impact on other outcomes such as mortality, nursing home admission rate, hospital readmission rate or quality of life (New South Wales Aged Care Assessment Program, 1996, para 3.65). Moreover control group clients, without the assistance of TCP, still appeared able to access community services reasonably quickly. As a result, it was not possible to demonstrate that TCP made a difference. A cost-effectiveness analysis was not carried out, but it seems likely that under these conditions the additional payment of prospective payments in the form of TCP would not prove cost-effective.

Although lacking a rigorous controlled evaluation, the Victoria TCP pilot was regarded by its evaluators as having achieved most of its objectives. The evaluators reported a reduction in inappropriate entry to residential care, and high levels of satisfaction among clients and carers. The project was also reported to have served as a catalyst for a number of other developments, including a GP Liaison Officer project and an extended coverage TCP operating in accident and emergency departments of public hospitals (Lincoln Gerontology Centre, 1996, p 116).

Drawing together the evaluations of the six State pilot projects, the national evaluation report distinguished the costs of TCPs from their outcomes for individual recipients and their outcomes for the organisations involved. The average national cost per client of TCPs was $1,529, just under $40 per day, with an average length of stay of 38.5 days. Marked variations in the total cost per client could, in a number of cases, be attributed to differences in the time that clients were on the programme. In New South Wales, for instance, clients remained on the TCP programme for an average of just over six weeks, while in Victoria, with a near identical daily cost, average length of stay was around three and a half weeks. Costs per day were about one third lower in Queensland, West Australia and South Australia, although this was not fully translated into lower total costs as length of stay was higher than in Victoria. The evaluation also reported that TCP was more cost-effective than the use of hostels or other forms of support (TCP National, 1996, pp 57-66). The national report also noted that TCP had facilitated access to a greater range and level of community services for hospital patients being discharged back home, and led to higher levels of user satisfaction with services (TCP National, 1996, pp 69-79). Hospital staff, ACATs and service providers all showed strong support for the programme. Evidence of the impact on mortality, nursing home admissions, hospital readmissions and functional status was, however, 'contradictory' (TCP National, 1996, pp 81-9).

Medicare Incentive Packages

The structure of the Medicare Agreements between the Commonwealth and State governments allows funds to be provided for special initiatives within the States' public hospital systems. Arrangements for the payment of special funds to encourage early discharge and facilitate treatment outside hospitals have been made under the last two Medicare agreements, 1988/

89 to 1991/92, and 1992/93 to 1997/98. In the first of these agreements, older patients were identified as the specific target population for 58 of the Medicare Incentive Packages, a number of which were specifically developed to encourage discharge planning by facilitating access to post-acute community care. Others covered orthogeriatric services and specialised assessment and rehabilitation services. As each represented a form of discretionary prospective payment, there is much that can be learnt about the operation of such payment mechanisms in the Australian context from their evaluation.

A major review of the effects of the MIP reported mixed success (Kasap and Associates, 1993). Of particular interest were projects in geriatric orthopaedics and rehabilitation, many of which led to increased costs with little measurable benefit and others which failed to achieve the projected savings. However, there were many other projects which did result in reduced length of hospital stay and reduced overall costs. A hallmark of these latter projects was that the MIP payments were accompanied by changes in hospital policy and practice and by domiciliary follow-up services. Other features of successful projects included the substitution of stays in less intensive 'step-down' units for high cost acute hospital beds for part of the in-patient treatment. A feature of those projects which did poorly was that MIP monies were simply treated as additional resources and were not used in ways which would have allowed the hospital to reduce other costs. This could occur, for example, where length of in-patient stay was reduced, but the savings achieved were used to admit additional patients. Successful projects, on the other hand, used the enhanced capacity provided by MIP payments to reduce in-patient costs and then made changes in the use of these resources to maintain the savings (Kasap and Associates, 1993, p 42).

A review of the first wave of MIP project evaluations showed that orthogeriatric units reduced bed day use by 20% to 30% of the average length of stay in hospital and rates of admission to residential long-term care in comparison to previous practice. Although there was a higher cost per remaining bed day, significant cost savings were achieved in the two projects in which an economic evaluation was conducted. The average reduction in length of stay was around eight days; this was accompanied by only a small increase in the use of existing community services. Reduced length of stay was achieved through better surgical procedures, more intensive rehabilitation and follow-up by hospital-based personnel (Howe, 1996, pp 29-30).

Medicare Incentive Payments continue to play a major role in the development of early discharge programmes in Queensland. Mitchell et al (1993) describe how MIPs were incorporated into a package of measures including a hospital Utilisation Review (a mechanism for ongoing review of the treatment and length of stay of individual hospital patients), a Community Based Discharge Management process, the contracting of services with community-based service providers, and ongoing monitoring and evaluation mechanisms. A before-and-after comparison indicated significant reductions in length of stay and readmission to hospital, as well as marked reductions in cost. For example, the readmission rate for medical/social patients fell from 18.8% to 4.9%. Approximately 60% of this group of patients were people aged 65 years or over who had been admitted for predominantly 'social factors' (ie, lack of support at home) (Mitchell et al, 1993, p 46).

An important consequence of the successful deployment of MIP funding has been the expansion of geriatric medical services (Howe, 1996, p 30). However, the limited use of MIP funding to purchase services from established community agencies suggests that there is still much to be learnt about the form that prospective payments should take. The evidence suggests that hospital staff have, by and large, opted to commit the funds internally, in the form of additional in-patient services, the direct provision of domiciliary follow-up teams or through outpatient clinics, rather than use these funds to purchase care from other organisations.

Organisational approaches

Assuming that additional assistance will be required, at least on a temporary basis, following a patient's discharge home from an acute care setting, the question arises as to how it should be best provided. Should post-acute care be provided by existing community-based service providers, or by a specialised team based in the hospital?

This question is hotly debated. For instance, the Council on the Ageing (Victoria) argues that so long as hospitals need incentives to take responsibility for post-acute care, it is better to promote the use of existing community based services than create new organisations or use hospital based services (COTA, 1994, pp 38-43). Providing financial incentives for hospitals to reduce length of stay and increase throughput has generally resulted in hospitals establishing their own early discharge or home care programmes: "this does not encourage links between existing community-based services, nor does it address the funding inadequacies faced by community-based services" (COTA, 1994, p 39). Drawing on the work of Adamson and Owen (1992), the report argues that extending hospital-based discharge services creates further problems for the integration of services and duplicates, from a hospital base, existing community care services. Caplan and Brown, who together are responsible for the Post-acute Care Service (PACS) operating from the Prince of Wales Hospital in Sydney, take the contrary position. They argue that, on balance, the advantage lies in outreaching from the hospital. It is vital to win the trust and agreement of the clinicians whose patients are to be involved in the scheme. For this reason nurses recruited from their wards have a large head start. Any post-acute care scheme must have a commitment to readmit, and a hospital-based team will more readily achieve this. A hospital-based team is more responsive to the dynamic, frequently shifting environment of the hospital. Finally, the development of a seamless service which starts in the pre-admission or outpatients clinic, through the admission to the post-discharge period needs a constantly available team (Caplan and Brown, 1996, pp 11-12).

Other reasons commonly advanced for hospitals developing their own post-acute care services, apart from cost arguments, are that the services do not exist in the community and would not be provided if the hospital did not provide them. It is also argued that where community support services do exist, they do not offer either the type or timeliness of support the hospital believes necessary; that they do not have the required level of skill; or that appropriate post-acute care services are outside the scope of the existing funding programme for community care.

A very recent innovation providing an important link between hospital and domiciliary services is currently being trialed at a number of locations in Australia. So-called 'quick response teams' operate through Accident and Emergency Departments, which are perhaps the most important single point of entry for older people to public hospitals (Stathers and Gonski, 1996). By intervening at the point of admission, not just at the point of discharge, quick response teams act to link individuals to community services and prevent a significant proportion of admissions to hospital that might otherwise have taken place (O'Grady et al, 1997).

Large-scale system redesign

Each of the interventions discussed above is intended to operate as an additional component within the existing financial and organisational infrastructure. Proposals for reform on a far larger scale have been developed by representatives of the Council of Australian Governments (COAG)[2].

The plans derive their approach from the principles set out in the National Competition Policy (Hilmer, 1993) and the experience of developments in healthcare financing such as GP fundholding in Britain and New Zealand and managed care in the USA. COAG originally proposed the replacement of over 60 different programmes, covering the entire health and community services fields, with just three streams of care: general care; acute care; and coordinated care (COAG, 1995a). These proposals, which in a single move would have had massive but unknown and unpredictable effects on the entire system of health and social care in Australia, were not implemented. Instead, the feasibility of the approach is to be tested by a series of large-scale trials, conducted under the direction of the Commonwealth government. The coordinated care stream, for people with complex care needs, is the first stream to be implemented. A series of 10 local trials, at least one in each State, is being conducted between 1997 and 1999 (Coopers & Lybrand, 1997). The trial populations cover frail older people, people with chronic mental health problems, specific disease groups (such as cancer) and aboriginal populations with high levels of health needs (Coopers & Lybrand, 1997).

The original proposals developed by COAG aimed to replace a variety of different funding streams, some of which include open-ended fee-for-service funding, with a more flexible system of pooled funding. This would be accessed by case managers responsible for the preparation of individual care plans for each enrolled client or patient. The approach originally proposed had much in common with that of managed competition, which has recently gained many influential advocates among senior health planning and research staff in Australia (Scotton, 1995). Preliminary plans envisaged case managers operating as budget holders, with an 'envelope of funds' equivalent to the pre-existing resources. These would be used to purchase a costed package of care and facilitate the substitution of a more efficient mix of services (COAG, 1995b). The purchase of services by case managers accessing pooled funding, it was argued, would overcome the problems of overlapping State and Commonwealth jurisdictions, because a single fund pool would be used in place of a series of carefully bounded programmes. The proposals were also seen as a way of removing the divide between public and private services, as budget holders would increasingly be in a position to force different providers to compete on the basis of output efficiency, rather than operate solely according to predetermined categories of programme funding. Most importantly, the reforms were intended to promote the coordination of different types of services, allowing acute hospitals to work closely with primary care and community support services.

Because the funding pool would not be open ended (as with most medical fee-for-service payments) but 'capped', it was argued that this would promote greater efficiency. Rather than being confined to using only those services for which there were financial payment programmes in place, case managers and those charged with administering the funds at local level would be able to use their pooled funds flexibly to get the best outcomes per dollar for each patient. For example, if an elderly patient requiring help after a stroke is discharged from hospital to her home, it is possible for her general practitioner to prescribe an almost unlimited amount of subsidised pharmaceuticals under existing funding arrangements. Although the judicious use of physiotherapy might be more cost-effective and prevent long-term disability, the patient would only be able to receive this if she had sufficient means to pay for it personally. Under the proposed pooled funding arrangements, funds which are currently only available for prescription drugs could instead be used to purchase paramedical services such as physiotherapy, or enhance community support provided in the person's home. The logic of capped pooled funding would provide a further incentive to substitute primary care and community services for more expensive hospital care whenever the clinical evidence suggested that this would not adversely affect outcomes for patients.

However, many in the health and community services systems, particularly in public services and the voluntary sector, have been concerned about the possible impact of the approach of managed competition. Possibly more surprising has been the hostile reaction of many of the medical profession, especially general practitioners. Part of the fear expressed is that the pooling of funding could result in a reduction of resources for primary care and community services, as previously dedicated resources are diverted to ease the budgetary problems experienced by hospitals and other areas of the health system. An associated anxiety, particularly on the part of non-medical community service providers, is that community care services will become 'medicalised' following a takeover by health service managers who control most trials. A third area of concern is that cheaper commercial providers may undercut the costs of publicly funded services and win contracts which would effectively put the existing providers out of business. The move from an open ended system of funding medical care through fee-for-service mechanisms, too, was regarded by many doctors as threatening their income and independence.

As a result of these misgivings, the trials as they have developed in practice appear to have taken on a more collaborative and less competitive approach. It proved difficult for many to believe that promoting competition for limited funding could enhance cooperation between services. Questions have also been asked about whether case management and pooled funding would actually enhance coordination between different services or simply increase competition. In establishing the trials, a more immediate question has been whether it would indeed prove possible to introduce a competitive model of service provision under the conditions required to induce services and programme managers to contribute existing funds to the pool. These questions remain unanswered at present. Each should, however, receive attention as part of the local and national evaluations of the coordinated care trials, which will run until at least the end of 1999 and in some cases at least until early 2000.

Two other initiatives also deserve some comment. The first concerns the attempt by some State governments, such as Victoria, to increase the integration of hospital and community care services by stipulating that close coordination will be a requirement of funding contracts (see, for example, DHS, 1998). The second concerns the development of Multi Purpose Services (MPS) that has taken place as a joint Commonwealth–State initiative in a number of smaller rural areas where the provision of separate hospital, residential care and community care services was not viable (DHSH, 1995). Despite the success of these initiatives, there have not been any attempts to try and replicate such services in more densely populated rural areas.

Conclusion: the uncertain future of of new care mixes

There is considerable interest among Australian policy makers and health system planners in promoting primary care solutions and breaking down the boundaries between hospital and extended home delivered care services. However it is not possible, at present, to speak of a single Australian model for integrating care services across the different sectors. This is because the different services have historically been organised and funded in fundamentally different ways; moreover, the current constitutional distinctions between Commonwealth and State responsibilities are likely to continue.

It is also clear that, at present, no single model for service integration has yet proven itself. Even if there were acceptance of a single 'best practice' model, any attempt to introduce systemic reform would be likely to face considerable opposition, as the likely winners and losers from any model that might be adopted would seek to influence its introduction. In assessing the likely success of future developments in this field it is also necessary to take into account the different structures and principles underpinning the healthcare system of each State and Territory government, as well as the considerable variation that exists between urban, rural and remote areas. There is also widespread recognition of the value of local flexibility in the provision of health and community services. There is, however, scope for the promotion of key elements of a common approach by the Commonwealth government acting together with the State and Territory governments, and it seems most likely that longer term changes will eventually be introduced in this way.

Despite the emphasis on improving integration between services, it would be wrong to assume that the existing system does not already allow at least some transitional use of community care services for older people discharged from hospital. Table 7.4 combines data from a recent study of post-acute care in two localities, Sutherland in New South Wales, and Gold Coast in South Eastern Queensland (Fine et al, 1997); a New South Wales study which reported on a general sample of 2,805 older people (65+) in Dubbo (McCallum et al, 1994); and a study from Bundoora in Melbourne, Victoria (Street, 1995), which traced service use and outcomes for 564 patients aged 65-plus, admitted to Preston and Northcot Community Hospital between December 1993 and April 1994, who had a hospital stay of four days or more.

Table 7.4: Summary of post-hospital service utilisation, calculated as percentage of older people (65+) discharged from hospital, Australia (1994-96)

Study (year)	Number 65+ discharged from hospital	Home nursing	Home care	Meals on wheels	Residential care
	N	%	%	%	%
Dubbo (1994)	263	12	2	4	2.4
Bundoora (1995)	564	26	26	17	17.4
Sutherland (1996)	3,702	11	1	2	1.3
Gold Coast (1996)*	5,168	23	0.1	n/a	4.4

Notes

(*) This sample includes patients referred to the nursing service using post-acute payments (PAP), a prospective payment scheme.

Percentages rounded to nearest whole number or decimal point.

To simplify the comparison, all post-hospital service users in Sutherland and the Gold Coast have been calculated as a percentage of those aged 65+. In practice, a significant minority of post-hospital service users in most studies are aged less than 65.

Those in the Bundoora study were, on average, more dependent on assistance than those in the Dubbo, Sutherland or Gold Coast samples. The high rate of admission to residential care in Bundoora, for example, reflects the fact that those involved were very disabled and more comparable to the high-need HACC population than to the general population of aged people admitted to an acute hospital.

The comparison presented in Table 7.4 shows that the use of post-hospital services overall was lowest in Sutherland and highest in the Bundoora case. Nonetheless, despite important differences, the order of magnitude of post-hospital service use is broadly similar in the Dubbo sample (McCallum et al, 1994) and in Sutherland. The use of home nursing on the Gold Coast approached that reported for the Bundoora sample. On the Gold Coast, approximately 11% of the total number of older people discharged from hospital were reported to have been classified as 'post-acute patients' for funding purposes.

Despite the different results reported, the figures for service utilisation show similar patterns in each of these studies. Home nursing, for example, was the most commonly used service for those discharged from hospital. Similarly, patterns of service usage for all services are roughly of the same order of magnitude. Unfortunately, with the exception of the figures concerning post-acute (PAP) funded patients on the Gold Coast, these results do not distinguish short term post-acute use from longer-term use of services; hospital discharge is simply a common reference point, either initiating a longer episode of use or simply being a break in an ongoing pattern of usage. What may seem a relatively modest flow of patients from the perspective of the hospital can be near overwhelming from the perspective of community services, with their limited staffing, less flexible funding and large proportion of long-term clients. Hospitals have long been a major source of referrals to community services and are often the single most important initiator of an episode of service to community care clients. The cost of providing patients with access to ongoing post-hospital services, often a relatively small cost in comparison to the cost of treatment in the hospital system, can be a major problem for community services. For this reason, access to additional resources to provide short-term care for post-acute patients is an issue of fundamental importance if community services are to be responsible for providing post-acute care without reducing the longer-term support required by their existing HACC clientele. How this seemingly inevitable development will finally take shape still remains very much an open question in Australia.

Notes

[1] This chapter draws on a number of reports written by the author and colleagues at the Social Policy Research Centre, University of New South Wales.

[2] COAG is a non-legislative forum in which the heads of the Commonwealth, State and Territory governments and a representative of local government are brought together on an irregular basis to discuss issues of common significance.

EIGHT

Conclusions: learning from abroad

Caroline Glendinning

Common themes and trends

The introduction to this book identified a number of common pressures which are currently influencing the funding and organisation of health and social welfare services for frail older people in post-industrial societies. To what extent are these pressures evoking similar changes across different societies in the scope and configuration of services for this growing sector of the population? To what extent are trends and developments characterised by a degree of convergence in the organisation and funding of long-term care services? For example, to what extent is health and welfare provision for frail older people increasingly financed by a mix of public and private funding? Are quasi-markets, in which alternative service providers compete with each other on price and quality and offer greater choice to older people needing support, a universal development in post-industrial welfare states? Or do historical differences in the welfare institutions and cultures of different countries shape and differentiate their responses to common demographic and economic pressures, thus constraining to a considerable extent the degree of convergence and similarity?

This chapter aims first of all to address these questions. It draws on the case studies of individual countries to summarise some main themes and trends in service developments. In doing so, it will identify areas of commonality between the different countries and also indicate some clear limitations to these common trends – the points at which different countries diverge from each other. What conclusions might be drawn from these experiences about the quality of life and citizenship of current and future cohorts of frail older people? The latter part of the chapter will focus on a number of key trends and developments and discuss their implications for the UK. To what extent might policy and service developments in the UK learn from the experiences of other countries?

Convergence and diversity in changing services for frail older people

Demographic trends, economic constraints on the continuing expansion of public sector funding and political trends away from public sector provision of services constitute common pressures for service development and change in the countries described in this book. However, these common pressures appear to exert different degrees of influence over welfare policy and service development or manifest themselves in different ways.

Responses to economic and demographic pressures

Economic and demographic pressures have undoubtedly played a major role in prompting large-scale reform and change, particularly where a lack of appropriate funding or service provision for long-term care has placed existing structures under considerable pressure. For example, growing pressures on taxation-funded health services or on sickness insurance schemes to finance long-term care services (as in Germany, Australia and The Netherlands) have prompted major policy and service changes. Increasing demands on means-tested social assistance budgets to fund institutional care for frail older people who have no other means of access to long-term care services have also prompted major reforms. This was particularly the case in the UK before the 1993 community care changes and in Germany before the introduction of the new care insurance scheme.

A key element of the drive to contain costs involves reducing pressures on medical services, hospitals and other healthcare institutions for the provision of nursing and personal care. All the countries described in this book are attempting to do this, to a greater or lesser extent (with the possible exception of some parts of Finland, where distance and sparse populations limit both the feasibility and the cost-effectiveness of cutting institutional provision and reinvesting in domiciliary services instead).

However, the actual responses of individual countries to these pressures are diverse and reflect, to a greater or lesser extent, rather more distinctive institutional and cultural traditions. For example, in countries with sickness insurance schemes, contractual and reimbursement mechanisms may make it easier to maintain a sharp separation between acute medical 'cure' services and long-term nursing and personal 'care' provision (as in Germany and The Netherlands); demands for increased expenditure on health services can be controlled simply by defining more clearly the boundaries between illness and long-term care and restricting insurance reimbursements to the former. Indeed, the new German care insurance scheme has not only relieved pressure on the sickness insurance scheme but effectively capped public spending on long-term care services as well.

Where there is an established tradition of health and/or social welfare services funded from taxation, these cost containment mechanisms are not available. Instead, a number of other strategies for containing costs are apparent.

Devolving and integrating budgets

One is the creation and devolution to local level of integrated budgets to cover most or all long-term care services – home help, personal care, home nursing, day care and respite and long-term care in institutions. The move to devolve responsibilities for the allocation and management of an integrated budget is perhaps most apparent in Finland, where central government subsidies for specific areas of municipal service provision have been replaced by a single block grant which municipalities themselves decide how to allocate between different services. The 1993 community care changes in the UK similarly brought together under the control of local authority social services departments the budgets for home help, day care and residential and nursing home care services (but not home nursing services). The development of integrated home care services in both Denmark and Finland has undoubtedly been facilitated by the fact that the budgets of local municipalities cover both primary and community health services and social welfare services. In The Netherlands, networks of service provider organisations have developed coordinated planning and service delivery strategies within the framework of single integrated budgets.

Integrated budgets offer a number of opportunities and advantages. First, they are easy to cap, particularly in comparison with individual budgets for particular services, which may be influenced by historical patterns of activity and professional interests. This, it has been argued, was one of the major imperatives behind the 1993 community care changes in the UK (Lewis and Glennerster, 1996). Second, devolved integrated budgets increase both the incentives and the opportunities for increasing the efficiency and cost–effectiveness of services. No longer can the scope and volume of some long-term services be altered without considering the implications for the budgets of other services. Overlaps and duplication of services also become both more visible and more easy to tackle. Services and the personnel who provide them can be more easily reallocated in response to changing needs and demands.

However, it is not always possible to create integrated budgets, particularly if responsibilities for controlling and allocating finance are divided between different levels of local, regional, and federal or national government. For example, in Denmark, the provision of hospital services is a county responsibility whereas primary and community health and social welfare services are all provided at local level. In Australia too, the respective responsibilities of State and Commonwealth governments for funding and providing services are integral elements of a carefully negotiated balance of power between State and Federal governments. Where such divisions of responsibility between different levels of government reflect important constitutional checks and balances (particularly checks on the powers of central or federal governments), it may be more difficult to create single, integrated, devolved budgets. Moreover, as anxieties in Australia have indicated, if devolved, integrated health and social welfare budgets include provision for acute hospital services, it may become necessary to 'ringfence' or protect elements of the budget specifically for spending on non–medical services.

Improving coordination across service boundaries

Nevertheless, even where budgets were not integrated, many of the countries described in this book had introduced mechanisms to improve the coordination and/or integration of services. This is a particular challenge in countries such as Australia, Germany and The Netherlands, with long traditions of 'mixed economies' of welfare in which independent, non–profit or commercial organisations have traditionally played a major role in providing domiciliary and/or institutional services. Trends towards increasing the coordination of services appear particularly common in relation to home care and home nursing services.

At an organisational level, mechanisms to increase the coordination of services include the creation of coordinated networks of provider organisations, integrated teams of home care workers and home nurses, financial incentives and initiatives to improve coordination between hospital and community services, and single, integrated teams which work with older people in both their own homes and in residential settings. Where budgetary and service provision responsibilities are divided between different levels of government, coordination between these levels is particularly important (as in the development of relationships between local municipalities and regional health authorities in The Netherlands and between nursing homes and community services in Australia).

At the level of individual service users, care management is a common mechanism for tailoring service inputs to the specific requirements of individual service users who have complex needs. Devolved budgets allow care or case managers to purchase packages of care from a number of different providers, using the most appropriate and cost-effective mix of services. Care management was a key element of the 'community care' changes in the UK, although care managers' budgets did not extend beyond the purchase of local authority social services. The Australian Coordinated Care Trials are also testing the effectiveness of care management. At its most extreme, the Dutch 'personal budget' experiment allows frail older people to act as purchasers themselves and maximises both their choice and control and cost-effectiveness. Again integrated budgets, whether devolved to local teams, care managers or frail older people themselves, can be easily capped, providing a major incentive to experiment with the substitution of services and maximise cost-effectiveness.

A further area in which major initiatives to increase coordination appear common is in relation to the boundaries between hospital and community-based services. Changes at this particular boundary partly reflect a redefinition of the role of hospitals, as described above, with their increasing emphasis on treating only acute illness on an in-patient basis. However, different funding streams, or service responsibilities which are divided between different professionals, organisations or tiers of government can create major barriers to the prompt discharge of older patients who may need considerable support and help for some time after illness or surgery. The problem here is the lack of leverage which acute hospitals have over the domiciliary services which older people need in order to support them at home after discharge. The initiatives in Denmark and Australia, in particular, illustrate a number of different strategies – fines for 'bed-blocking', prospective payments to enable hospital-based personnel to purchase community services, and liaison workers to provide continuity during the discharge process – for addressing this particular boundary. The Netherlands has also created initiatives to avoid hospital 'bed-blocking' and improve continuity between hospital and home-based services for frail older people.

Even more challenging is the boundary between institutional care in nursing and residential homes, and services for very frail older people in their own homes. The experiments in Denmark and The Netherlands have attempted in a number of different ways to break down this particular barrier and create greater commonality in the funding, organisation and delivery of services across these two settings. These initiatives aim to create greater flexibility and continuity for frail older people who may need to spend intermittent spells in nursing or residential homes (for example, for convalescence after illness or to give family carers a break). They also appear to offer opportunities to develop the more intensive services, which might normally be associated with institutional care, for frail older people living in their own homes and hence enable them to avoid admission to a residential or nursing home.

None of the countries described in this book has extended the purchasing and coordination of health and social care services into the areas of primary or specialist medical services, alongside long-term nursing and personal care services. This broader approach to purchasing and coordinating services for frail older people features in a number of demonstration projects in the United States (Robinson and Steiner, 1998, pp 14-15). It is far from clear whether the various systems of funding primary and hospital medical services in the countries described here could be extended to a full managed care approach in the future.

From public to private responsibilities

To what extent have the countries described in this book sought to contain public expenditure by shifting responsibilities for the funding or provision of long-term care services to frail older people themselves and their families? This does appear to have occurred, although the extent, the nature and the visibility of this public-to-private shift are highly variable. First, in both the UK and Germany, family members play a major role in the care of frail older people: in the UK, this has been actively encouraged by successive governments for almost two decades; in Germany, the care insurance cash payment option is widely believed to act as an incentive for family-based care for frail older people. The limited personal budget experiment in The Netherlands may also have sustained some informal care arrangements.

The introduction of charges for services also effectively shifts the balance of responsibility for funding from public to private purses. This has been particularly marked in the UK, in relation to both home care, residential home and nursing home services, and in Finland, where charges also extend to home nursing and other community-based health services. In both countries, income from service charges is expected to generate a considerable proportion of the total service budget.

However, the introduction of user charges for collectively funded services can itself facilitate or encourage the further 'privatisation' of long-term care. In Finland, for example, the widespread introduction of charges for municipal services has reduced the gap between private and public services, so far as service users are concerned. If private providers can match the quality of municipal services, then differential cost factors will provide less and less of a barrier to the purchase of services in the private market. In Denmark, the introduction of charges as a means of equalising public and private provision has been much more selective and has occurred only in relation to home cleaning and other domestic services, with municipalities withdrawing cleaning from the range of home care services they provide and/or requiring those who want these services to pay for them. In Germany, any assistance needed with household tasks is discounted in the assessment for care insurance, which focuses only on personal care and supervision needs. In the UK too, local authority home care services have increasingly withdrawn from offering domestic help and now provide only personal care. It therefore appears that help with domestic and household tasks are increasingly excluded from state funded or subsidised welfare services and older people have to purchase this from either public or private suppliers.

The role of quasi-markets in the development of long-term care services

To what extent have quasi-markets played a major role in these changing patterns of long-term care? The evidence from the countries in this book is mixed. In the UK, quasi-markets have been central to the development of health and social care services, although they have developed more extensively in the institutional than the domiciliary social care sector and medical and home nursing care is still provided from within the NHS. In Germany, the resources now available through the care insurance scheme (and the associated legislation which gives preference to independent over public provider organisations) could provide a stimulus to the development of a more competitive and responsive market. However, the massive preference shown by care insurance beneficiaries for the cash rather than the 'in kind' service option is likely to restrict this potential demand-side factor. In contrast, long-term care services in Australia have traditionally always been provided through a mix of public, private, commercial and non-profit organisations.

Moreover, developments in a number of countries illustrate the practical and political limitations to quasi-markets in long-term care, particularly the tensions between, on the one hand, using market mechanisms to improve quality, increase choice and drive down costs and, on the other hand, increasing the coherence and coordination of services. The Australian initiatives described in Chapter Seven aim to reduce some of the problems arising from a long tradition of providing both institutional and home care services through a mixture of public, private and voluntary organisations. In both The Netherlands and Denmark too, very considerable caution has been exercised in encouraging 'mixed economies' of welfare, even within the highly circumscribed arena of home care services. Private provider organisations have been given only limited encouragement to enter into market competition with traditional public home care services, because of the increased difficulties in coordinating services and higher risk of fragmentation. In Denmark, in particular, the contracting out of home care services is regarded as a major threat to the integrated area and joint operation teams which have developed to bridge the traditional fragmentation between home care and home nursing services and between domiciliary services and institutional care.

The operation of quasi-markets also requires that 'care'-related services are commodified so that contracts can be issued and reimbursement arranged. This can restrict the discretion and responsiveness which service providers can exercise. In Denmark, for example, contracting out has also been opposed because it reduces opportunities for the service providers who are in day to day contact with frail older people to respond quickly and flexibly to changes in their needs.

Trends in the governance and management of long-term care

Despite the sometimes substantial differences between the different countries described in this book, some broad common trends and themes can nevertheless be discerned. These trends can be brought together to construct a theoretical model. No single country exhibits all the characteristics to the maximum possible degree and it is important not to overlook the distinctive patterns and traditions of different countries which shape and give character to their responses to the new challenges of long-term care. Nor is the following description intended to imply a determinism whereby welfare states will all eventually converge towards a single model. Nevertheless, a number of broad commonalities do seem to underlie a range of apparently diverse developments. Most importantly, these common themes also help to indicate some likely consequences for the quality of life of frail older people and for their citizenship of the societies to which they have contributed – and continue to – contribute.

Many of the trends described in this book reflect a diminution of professional and bureaucratic influences in shaping services and an increase in managerialism, particularly that associated with the New Public Management (Osborne and Gaebler, 1992). The traditional segmentation of medical, nursing and social care services largely reflects different professional interests. Hierarchical service sectors tended to reflect and reinforce these professional boundaries and interests. In contrast, the influence of the New Public Management movement is prompting the search for more efficient and accountable organisational structures to replace large scale bureaucratic models (Fine, 1996). Consistent with this trend, the development of long-term care services is tending to take place within local, devolved organisational frameworks, in which the emphasis is on the horizontal coordination and integration of multiple services for a locality, rather than the provision of services for the clientele of a particular professional group. Developments in Denmark, Australia and Finland have taken place within traditional constitutional frameworks of devolved responsibility. The Netherlands has placed considerable emphasis on the local coordination of long-term care services. The 1993 community care changes in the UK effectively devolved responsibility for the funding and purchasing of institutional care from the national social security system to local authority social services departments, where these services could be better integrated with the home and community services which local authorities were already providing. At the most extreme is the devolution of responsibility for coordinating services to individual service users. Arguably the German care insurance and the Dutch personal budget pilot schemes do this, through their emphasis on individual benefit entitlements and the absence of brokerage or care management services.

A second common theme is the growing use of capped single or integrated budgets, for purchasing a whole range of long-term care services. These allow costs to be contained by central government or the main funding organisations; they also offer opportunities and incentives for service substitutions and increased efficiency. The development of coordinated service networks in The Netherlands and integrated local area teams in Denmark demonstrate how these opportunities can be maximised. Again, integrated budgets can be introduced at the level of individual service users, as in the debates in Finland about the possible introduction of vouchers for long-term care services.

Thirdly, market-derived mechanisms, such as the separation between purchasers and provider organisations, outcome-based contracting and increasing choices for users are increasingly shaping the regulation and supply of services. The widespread introduction of such mechanisms enables boundaries to be removed between public and private sector providers of services and forces public sector organisations (which may hitherto have maintained a monopoly over the supply of services) to compete with other providers. Conversely, the managerial and regulatory frameworks associated with the purchase of services from private providers in a 'mixed economy' of welfare are also increasingly regulating the supply of public sector services.

The implications for older people

These trends have a number of important implications for current and future cohorts of frail older people.

First, the creation of capped budgets from which publicly-funded long-term care services are provided is likely to assign increasing importance to the role of assessment in targeting services at the frailest older people or those at greatest risk. This is already apparent, for example, in the standard 'care dependency' guidelines for the German care insurance assessment, the importance of assessment in the UK 'community care' changes, the introduction of specialised, multi-disciplinary Aged Care Assessment Teams in Australia and the use of independent local or regional agencies to carry out assessments in The Netherlands on behalf of local governments and regional health insurance firms. Growing pressures on these capped budgets may increasingly restrict publicly-funded services only to those older people at the highest levels of dependency or at the most serious risk of harm. Opportunities for rehabilitation or preventative service interventions may increasingly be overlooked; older people who fall outside current assessment guidelines may experience a widening 'dependency trap', in which the disadvantages of not receiving care-related benefits or services far outweigh any advantages conferred by marginally better health or greater independence.

Second, trends in the funding and organisation of long-term care services may reinforce other trends in the material circumstances of frail older people. The expectations of future generations of older people who have benefited from extensive state welfare provision during their adult lives are likely to continue to grow. Many older people are also likely to enter retirement in good health and with levels of private pensions and private health insurance which will exclude them from increasingly residual state provision. On the other hand, a substantial minority of older people will take with them into later life levels of disadvantage which they experienced during their adult working lives. Gender, ethnicity and nationality, and access to training and secure employment in adulthood are all likely to have an increasing impact on life chances and material circumstances in old age.

Consequently, future generations of older people are likely to be increasingly differentiated between those who are able to exercise choice in 'quasi-markets' of long-term care services; and those who lack either the material or personal resources to choose, purchase and control the services they need.

The foundations of this emerging social division of old age are already apparent. First, for example, there has been concern in Germany that social and recreational activities will be excluded from the services provided by institutions for care insurance beneficiaries, because some older people will be unable to afford to purchase these extra services privately. The exclusion of domestic help from home care services in many countries also disadvantages those older people who cannot afford to purchase them privately. More generally, behaving as a 'consumer' of long-term care services requires a degree of literacy, confidence and competence. Frail older people whose first language is not that of their country of residence, who are confused or who do not have relatives to act on their behalf are likely to be particularly disadvantaged 'consumers'. For example, although the new German care insurance scheme confers clear benefit entitlements on frail older people, there is concern about the serious lack of information, advice, brokerage and care management services to help older people negotiate with formal service provider organisations.

The trend towards the devolution of responsibility for planning and coordinating long-term care services to local levels raises important questions about equity and citizenship. To what extent do older people in different localities experience different conditions of access to services or different patterns of provision? To what extent are these differences reflected in different choices, options or outcomes? What, if any, is the role of national governments in regulating minimum levels of provision or quality of services? Already these questions have been raised in the UK, in relation to local variations in conditions of access to NHS and local authority long-term care services and in relation to different local policies for charging for services. They are also a major issue in Finland, where the replacement of municipal subsidies by single block grants has led central government to relinquish much of its role in regulating the production of health and social care services by local municipalities, to the extent that some younger disabled people are taking legal actions to establish rights to municipal services.

However, devolved responsibilities for planning and providing services do not necessarily threaten the citizenship rights of frail older people. In Denmark, for example, strong traditions of local autonomy and the variable implementation of new service initiatives appear to be allowing the tailoring of services to local needs without compromising the rights of older people. However, even within a future of increasingly devolved local responsibilities for long-term care, the evidence from the countries described in this book suggest that there is still an important role for overarching regulatory frameworks. Moreover, it could be argued that the trend away from hierarchical professional and bureaucratic organisations to local coordinated networks as the main framework for delivering services makes such regulatory frameworks even more vital, in order to ensure that older people have the equal access to services on which social citizenship (Plant, 1992) is founded. These frameworks could include regulating the quality of services, both those which are purchased privately by more affluent or socially independent older people and those which are publicly funded. The development of benchmarking in The Netherlands to regulate the outputs, quality and pricing of both independent and statutory service providers is one possible example. A second example is the encouragement and support given by both the Danish and Dutch governments to the formal evaluation of local experimental and pilot projects. With this support, wider lessons can be learned and the benefits of local innovations distributed more widely.

The development of long-term care services for frail older people in Britain

Finally, what lessons can be learned from these varied experiences about the development of health and social care services for frail older people in the UK? As has been argued above, political and cultural traditions and established institutional structures limit the extent to which policy and practices can simply be modelled on developments in other countries. Nevertheless, there are a number of aspects of policy and service development from other countries which might offer useful broad objectives, if not detailed blueprints, for the UK.

First, in many areas of Finland, The Netherlands and Denmark, personal home care and home nursing services are closely aligned or are integrated into single teams with a single management structure and, in some instances, an integrated budget and common training as well. In most parts of the UK, the separate funding streams and management structures of NHS and local authority services make this impossible. Only in Northern Ireland, where health and social services are funded from a single revenue stream and where community health and social welfare services are often provided from the same community trust provider organisation, is such integration currently possible. Moreover, NHS policies during the 1990s have emphasised the closer alignment of home nursing services with general practice and primary medical services, first through GP fundholders' purchasing of home nursing and latterly through the involvement of community health services in the new Primary Care Groups which are to replace fundholding (DoH, 1997c).

At the operational level of 'front–line' services, relationships between social services home care staff and community nurses are already often close. However, this often depends largely on the individuals involved and rarely extends beyond coordination over service delivery to broader strategic issues of service planning (Rummery and Glendinning, 1997a; Glendinning and Rummery, 1998). Yet there would seem to be considerable scope for integrating more closely the home and personal care services provided by local authorities and the home nursing services provided through the NHS – and preferably within the framework of a single budget. The systematic integration of home care and home nursing teams would have considerably greater potential for reducing overlaps and duplication of services, could facilitate greater flexibility in providing the most appropriate type of input (rather than the service which simply happens to be available), could improve coordination when more than one type of service is needed and would ensure closer continuity when needs change and different service inputs are required. It would reduce one of the major areas of weakness in the 1993 'community care' changes – the lack of purchasing leverage which local authority social services department care managers have over home nursing and other services funded and provided by NHS organisations. Above all, reducing fragmentation and improving continuity in the provision of personal, sometimes highly intimate care, is likely to be valued very highly by older service users and their families.

Integrating home care and home nursing services could also provide a sound basis for a second area of service development – reducing the boundaries between domiciliary services and those provided in residential and nursing homes. Both Danish and Dutch service initiatives have aimed explicitly to reduce admissions to residential and nursing homes. Appropriately adapted, sheltered housing for frail older people has been a key element of these initiatives; closely coordinated or integrated multi-disciplinary domiciliary care services constitute the other important element. At present in the UK, there is very little flexibility between domiciliary and institutional care, apart from the use of residential and nursing homes for respite care and, sometimes, day care. However, even here, the two sectors are governed by different funding streams, users are subject to different means-testing and charging regimes and there is very unlikely to be any continuity in staffing across the two sectors.

Integrated home nursing and personal care services could offer opportunities for greater flexibility and responsiveness in the provision of very intensive levels of support, particularly in relation to the provision of support at evenings, night-times and weekends. Closer links would also need to develop with the largely private residential and nursing home sector, in order to bring them into new coordinating and partnership relationships. In many areas, good relationships have developed between local authority social services purchasers and private nursing and residential homes, but these have not involved either the purchasers or the providers of NHS nursing services. The substantial independent sector residential and nursing home market which has developed in the UK over the past 15 years may, together with the continuing divisions between NHS and local authority funding and services, constitute a very considerable barrier to closer integration. This may therefore be one area of potential service development which is rendered particularly problematic by the widespread development of quasi-markets and private sector provision.

Coordinating more closely or integrating home care and home nursing services could contribute to easing movement across another service boundary – that between acute hospital and community-based services. In most of the countries in this book (including the UK), growing demands for long-term care services have caused tighter boundaries to be drawn around hospital and specialist medical services. The result is a more rigid division between the treatment of acute illness and the provision of longer-term nursing and personal care. Yet the tightening of this boundary has created more problems, particularly in ensuring that appropriate levels of coordinated services can be provided for frail older people to support their early discharge or prevent their admission to hospital because appropriate domiciliary services are not available. Integrated domiciliary care teams, which included both nursing and personal care services, would make the arrangement of post-discharge care considerably easier. Other initiatives might include involving community-based staff in hospital discharge planning, and the various incentives and prospective payment initiatives in Australia to enable hospital-based staff to arrange appropriate post-discharge support.

A final, but nevertheless important set of boundaries to which attention needs to be drawn are those between health, social services and housing for older people. Public policies in Denmark and The Netherlands, in particular, assume that appropriate housing provision is an integral part of community care services and a key element in helping frail older people to maintain their independence. Community alarm schemes, aids and adaptations, specialised supported housing and home improvement agencies (sometimes called 'care and repair' schemes) which use the equity invested in privately owned housing to fund essential repairs and refurbishment all have a role to play in preventing admission to residential care, facilitating discharge from hospital after illness and reducing the levels of other services inputs such as home care. Indeed, there may be opportunities for overall increases in cost-effectiveness, if an appropriately adapted home environment leads to a reduction in substantial inputs of home care and other services.

However, changes in the role of housing authorities, the 'Right-to-Buy' provisions for local authority tenants and constraints on public capital investment have together dramatically reduced the availability of social housing, so that local authorities and other housing agencies are now struggling to cope with the rising numbers of people with special needs living in the community (Audit Commission, 1998). The responsibilities of housing authorities to collaborate in the joint commissioning of services is unclear. Funding for the housing aspects of community care is currently fragmented between a number of central and local government departments and is poorly targeted (or entirely untargeted) on those who need it (Audit Commission, 1998, p 74). Moreover, proposed changes to the system of housing benefit (subsidies to low-income owners or tenants in respect of their housing costs) threaten to exclude from the scheme the costs of housing-related care and support services. Clarification of responsibilities, a more rational funding framework and clear incentives for housing agencies to collaborate with other purchasers and providers of health and care services for frail older people are all urgently required.

The boundaries between NHS and local authority services have become more clearly and rigidly drawn over the past 50 years (Hudson, 1998). However, new policy initiatives offer opportunities to begin breaking down some of these distinctions, creating closer relationships at both strategic and operational levels, and possibly even the opportunity to experiment with 'pooled' budget arrangements. Eleven Health Action Zones in different parts of England will, between 1998 and 2005, focus on breaking down existing barriers and boundaries to improve the effectiveness of services. Pilot projects aimed at improving the coordination of services for older people – and the involvement of older people in those services – will also begin during 1998, under the 'Better Government for Older People' initiative. These initiatives will offer opportunities to experiment with some of the ideas described in this book.

Bibliography

Adamson, L. and Owen, A. (1992) 'Sharing the burden of shorter stays', in F. Baum, D. Fry and I. Lenny (eds) *Community health policy and practice in Australia*, Sydney: Pluto Press.

AIHW (Australian Institute of Health and Welfare) (1994a) *Health Expenditure Bulletin No 10*, December.

AIHW (1994b) *Health Expenditure Bulletin No 9*, November.

AIHW (1995) *Australia's welfare, services and assistance 1995*, Canberra: AGPS.

AIHW (1997) *Australia's welfare, services and assistance 1997*, Canberra: AGPS.

Alban, A., Boll Hansen, E., Christiansen, U. (1988) *Opgave glidning mellem sygehuse og kommuner*, Copenhagen: Danish Institute for Local Government Research (AKF) and Danish Institute for Health Services Research and Development (DSI).

Alber, J. (1995) 'A framework for the comparative study of social services', *Journal of European Social Policy*, vol 5, no 2, pp 131-49.

Alber, J. (1996) 'The debate about long-term care reform in Germany', in OECD Social Policy Studies, No 19, *Caring for frail elderly people*, Paris: OECD, pp 261-78.

Allemeyer, J. (1994a) 'Die Chance zu Reformen', *Altenheim*, vol 7, pp 490-9.

Allemeyer, J. (1994b) 'Die Pflegeversicherung', *Altenpflege*, vol 5, pp 315-20.

Allen, I., Hogg, D. and Peace, S. (1992) *Elderly people: Choice, participation and satisfaction*, London: Policy Studies Institute.

Alter, C. and Hage, J. (1993) *Organisations working together*, Newbury Park, Ca: Sage.

Anker, J. and Kock-Nielsen, I. (1995) *Det frivillige arbejde*, Copenhagen: Danish National Institute of Social Research (SFI).

Antikainen, E. and Vaarama, M. (1995) *Kotihoidon tuesta omaishoidon tukeen*, Jyvaskyla: Stakes, Raportteja 172, Gummerus Kirjapaino Oy (abstract).

Anttonen, A. and Sipilä, J. (1996) 'European social care services: is it possible to identify models?', *Journal of European Social Policy*, vol 6, no 2, pp 87-100.

Association of County Councils and National Association of Municipalities (1991) *Ventepatienter på sygehusene*, Copenhagen.

Atkin, K. (1998) 'Ageing in a multi-racial Britain: demography, policy and practice', in M. Bernard and J. Phillips (eds) *The social policy of old age*, London: Centre for Policy on Ageing.

Audit Commission (1992) *Community care: Managing the cascade of change*, London: HMSO.

Audit Commission (1995) *United they stand: Coordinating care for elderly patients with hip fracture*, London: HMSO.

Audit Commission (1996) *Balancing the care equation*, London: HMSO.

Audit Commission (1997) *The coming of age: Improving care services for older people*, London: The Audit Commission.

Audit Commission (1998) *Home alone*, London: Audit Commission.

Baldock, J. and Evers, A. (1991a) 'Citizenship and frail older people: changing patterns of provision in Europe', in N. Manning (ed) *Social policy review 1990-91*, Harlow: Longman.

Baldock, J. and Evers A. (1991b) 'Concluding remarks on the significance of the innovations', in R. Kraan (ed) *Care for the elderly: Significant innovations in three European countries*, Boulder, Colorado: Westview Press, pp 186-202.

Baldock, J. and Evers, A. (1992) 'Innovations in care for the elderly: the cutting edge of change for social welfare systems. Examples from Sweden, the Netherlands and the United Kingdom', *Ageing and Society*, vol 12, no 3, pp 289-312.

Baldock, J. and Ungerson, C. (1994) *Becoming consumers of community care*, York: Joseph Rowntree Foundation.

Baldwin, S. and Lunt, N. (1996) *Charging ahead: The development of local authority charging policies for community care*, Bristol: The Policy Press.

Barnes, M. (1997) *Care, communities and citizens*, Harlow,: Longman.

BAS (Bundesministerium für Arbeit und Sozialordnung) (1998) *Bericht über die Entwicklung der Pflegeversicherung*, January, Bonn: BAS.

Berman, P., Hunter, D. and McMahon, L. (1990) 'Keep it integrated', *Health Services Journal*, vol 5, pp 996-7.

Bewley, C. and Glendinning, C. (1994) *Involving disabled people in community care planning*, York: Joseph Rowntree Foundation.

Boll Hansen, E. (1997) *The state of the debate on social protection for dependency in old age in Denmark*, Copenhagen: Danish Institute of Local Government Research (AKF).

Boll Hansen, E. and Platz, M. (1995a) *Kommunernes til ældre – kommenteret tabelsamling*, Copenhagen: Danish National Institute of Social Research (SFI) and Danish Institute of Local Government Research (AKF).

Boll Hansen, E. and Platz, M. (1995b) *80-100 åriges levekår – en interviewundersrgelse blandt ældre I 75 kommuner*, Copenhagen: Danish National Institute of Social Research (SFI) and Danish Institute of Local Government Research (AKF).

Boll Hansen, E. and Platz, M. (1996) *Gamle danskere – nogle uddybende analyser af de 80-100 åriges levevilkår*, Copenhagen: Danish National Institute of Social Research (SFI 96.24) and Danish Institute of Local Government Research (AKF).

Boll Hansen, E. and Werborg, R. (1984a) *Døgnhjemmeplejen i Næstved I. Ressourcer og aktiviteter*, Copenhagen: Danish Institute of Local Government Research (AKF).

Boll Hansen, E. and Werborg, R. (1984b) *Døgnhjemmeplejen i Næstved II. Virkninger og konomi*, Copenhagen: Danish Institute of Local Government Research (AKF).

Boll Hansen, E. and Werborg, R. (1985) *Hjemmesygepleje hele døgnet. Et forsøg på Amager*, Copenhagen: Danish Institute of Local Government Research (AKF).

Boll Hansen, E., Jordal-Jørgensen, J. and Koch, A. (1991) *Fra plejehjem til hjemmepleje*, Copenhagen: Danish Institute of Local Government Research (AKF).

Boll Hansen, E., Eskelinen, L., Sejr, T. and Wagner, L. (1997) *Ældrevenlige behandlingsforløb – en analyse af fem indsatstyper*, Copenhagen: Danish Institute of Local Government Research (AKF) and Danish Institute for Health Services Research and Development (DSI).

Boot, J.M. and Knapen, M.H.J.M. (1996) *De Nederlandse gezondheidszorg*, Utrecht: Het Spectrum.

Bradshaw, J. and Gibbs, I. (1988) 'Dependency and its relationship to the assessment of care needs of elderly people', *British Journal of Social Work*, vol 8, no 4, pp 577-92.

Bynoe, I. (1996) *Beyond the Citizen's Charter*, London: Institute for Public Policy Research.

Cantor, M.H. (1980) 'The informal support system: its relevance in the lives of the elderly', in E.F. Borgatta and N.G. McCluskey (eds) *Aging and society: Current research and policy perspectives*, Beverly Hills, Ca: Sage, pp 131-45.

Caplan, G.A. and Brown, A. (1996) 'Post-acute care', Prince of Wales Hospital, Randwick, Sydney, NSW: Prince of Wales Hospital.

Castles, F. (1993) *Families of nations*, Aldershot: Dartmouth.

Chetwynd, M., Ritchie, J., Reith, L. and Howard, M. (1996) *The cost of care: The impact of charging policy on the lives of disabled people*, Bristol: The Policy Press.

Clarke, P. and Bowling, A. (1990) 'The quality of everyday life in long stay institutions for the elderly', *Social Science and Medicine*, vol 3, no 4, pp 1201-10.

Clasen, J. (1994) 'Social security – the core of the German employment-centred social state', in J. Clasen and R. Freeman (eds) *Social policy in Germany*, London: Harvester Wheatsheaf, pp 61-82.

COAG (Council of Australian Governments) (1995a) *Health and community services: Meeting people's needs better*, Discussion Paper, Canberra: Commonwealth Department of Human Services and Health.

COAG (1995b) *Call for expressions of interest in conducting trials in coordinated care*, Canberra: Commonwealth Department of Human Services and Health.

Coolen, J. (1993) *Changing care for the elderly in the Netherlands: Experiences and research findings from policy experiments*, Assen/Maastricht:Van Gorcum.

Coolen, J. (1994) 'Effects of policy experiments in long-term care: some empirical findings from the Netherlands', *Research in the Sociology of Health Care*, JAI Press Inc, vol 11, pp 69-88.

Coolen, J. (1997) 'Integrated health care for chronically disabled elderly people', in J. Kronenfeld (ed) *Research in the sociology of health care*, vol 14, Greenwich: JAI Press.

Coopers & Lybrand (1997) *Evaluation framework. Evaluation of coordinated care trials*, Canberra: Commonwealth Department of Health and Family Services.

Corden, A. (1992) 'Geographical development of the long-term care market for elderly people', *Transactions of the Institute of British Geographers*, vol 17, pp 80-94.

COTA (Council on the Ageing) Victoria (1994) *Removing the boundaries: Hospital discharge practices and older people returning to the community*, Melbourne.

Daatland, S.O. (ed) (1997) *De siste årene. Eldreomsorg i Scandinavia 1960-95*, NOVA-rapport 22/1997, Oslo: Norsk Institutt for Forskning om Opvekst Velferd og Aldring.

Danish Nurses' Organisation (1989) *Hjemmesygeplejen i en omstillingstid*, Copenhagen.

Danish Nurses' Organisation (1991) *Længst muligt i eget hjem – den integrerede ordning*, Copenhagen.

Davis, A., Ellis, K. and Rummery, K. (1997) *Access to assessment: Perspectives of practitioners, disabled people and carers*, Bristol: The Policy Press.

DCS (Department of Community Services) (1986) *Nursing homes and hostels review*, Canberra: AGPS.

DHFS (Department of Health and Family Services) (1996) *Draft guidelines for discharge planning and post discharge care*, Canberra: Health Services Outcomes Branch, Canberra.

DHHCS (Department of Health, Housing and Community Services) (1991) *Aged care reform strategy mid term review 1990-91*, Canberra: AGPS.

DHS (Department of Human Services) Victoria, Northern Metropolitan Region (1998) *Primary care redevelopment. Background Paper 4,* Fitzroy, Victoria.

DHSH (Department of Human Services and Health) (1994) *Annual Report 1993-94,* Canberra: AGPS.

DHSH (1995) *The efficiency and effectiveness review of the home and community care program. Final Report,* Aged and Community Care Division, Service Development and Evaluation Reports No 18, Canberra: AGPS.

Diba, R. (1996) *Meeting the costs of continuing care: Public views and perceptions,* York: Joseph Rowntree Foundation.

Dieck, M. (1990) 'Politics for elderly people in the FRG', in A. Jamieson and R. Illsley (eds) *Contrasting European policies for the care of older people,* Aldershot: Gower, pp 95-119.

Dieck, M. (1994) 'Reforming against the grain: long-term care in Germany', in R. Page and J. Baldock (eds) *Social Policy Review 6,* University of Kent: Social Policy Association, pp 253-66.

Dieck, M. and Garms-Homolová, V. (1991) 'Home-care services in the Federal Republic of Germany', in A. Jamieson (ed) *Home care for older people in Europe,* Oxford: Oxford University Press, pp 118-56.

DoH (Department of Health) (1995) *NHS responsibilities for meeting continuing health care needs,* HSG(95)8, London: HMSO.

DoH (1997a) *Community care statistics 1997: Residential personal social services for adults, England,* London: HMSO.

DoH (1997b) *Health action zones: Invitation to bid,* EL97(65), London: HMSO.

DoH (1997c) *The new NHS: Modern, dependable,* London: HMSO.

DoH/SSI (Social Services Inspectorate)/Scottish Office SWSG (Social Work Services Group) (1991a) *Care management and assessment: Managers' guide,* London: HMSO.

DoH/SSI/Scottish Office SWSG (1991b) *Care management and assessment: Practitioners' guide,* London: HMSO.

Donnelly, C., Kelly, J., Stewart, K. and Armstrong, S. (1995) *Community home nursing groups. Report on the Australian Community Nursing Casemix Development Project*, North Sydney: NSW Health Department.

Dudey, S. (1991) 'Verteilungswirkungen einer Gesetzlichen Pflegeversicherung', *Wirtschaftsdienst*, vol VII, pp 356-9.

Eager, K. (1996) 'Classification systems for psychiatric, sub-acute and non-acute services: implications for health information management', Preliminary Paper for the SNAP Project, University of Wollongong: Centre for Health Services Development.

Elder Commission (1980) *Aldersforandringer, ældrepolitikkens grundlag*, 1, delrapport, Copenhagen.

Elder Commission (1981) *De ældres vilkår*, 2, delrapport, Copenhagen.

Elder Commission (1982) *Sammenhæng i ældre politikken*, Afsluttende og 3, delrapport, Copenhagen.

Ellis, K. (1995) 'Burdensome parents: reciprocity, rationing and needs assessment', in H. Dean (ed) *Parents' duties, children's debts*, Aldershot: Arena.

Esping Andersen, G. (1990) *The three worlds of welfare capitalism*, Cambridge: Polity Press.

Estes, C. (1986) 'The aging enterprise: in whose interests?', *International Journal of Health Services*, vol 16, pp 243-51.

Evers, A. (1993) 'The welfare mix approach: understanding the pluralism of welfare systems', in A. Evers and I. Svetlik (eds) *Balancing pluralism*, Vienna: European Centre for Social Welfare Policy and Research, pp 3-22.

Evers, A. (1995) 'Die Pflegeversicherung – ein mixtum compositum im Prozeß der politischen Umsetzung', *Sozialer Fortschritt*, vol 2, pp 23-8.

Evers, A. (1996) 'The new Long Term Care Insurance in Germany: characteristics, consequences and perspectives', in T. Harding, B. Meredith and G. Wistow (eds) *Options for long term care: Economic, social and ethical choices*, London: HMSO, pp 122-35.

Evers, A., Pijl, M. and Ungerson, C. (eds) (1994) *Payments for care*, Aldershot: Avebury and Vienna: European Centre.

Falkingham, J. (1998) 'Financial (in)security in later life', in M. Bernard and J. Phillips (eds) *The social policy of old age*, London: Centre for Policy on Ageing.

Felbo, O. and Søland, AM. (1996) *Ældre og sundhedsvæsenet – hvordan gør vi det bedre?*, Copenhagen: Ældresagen/DanAge and Akademisk Forlag.

Fine, M.D. (1995a) 'Community based services and the fragmentation of provision', *Australian Journal of Social Issues*, vol 30, no 2, pp 143-61.

Fine, M.D. (1995b) 'Innovation and change in long term care: challenges of new models of support', in P. Saunders (ed) *Social policy and Northern Australia: National policies and local issues*, Reports and Proceedings 120, Sydney: Social Policy Research Centre.

Fine, M. (1995c) *The changing mix of welfare in health care and community support*, Discussion Paper 61, Sydney: Social Policy Research Centre.

Fine, M.D. (1996) *Competition or cooperation? Models for the development of integrated community care services in Australia*, Paper presented to the Annual Conference of the Australia/New Zealand Association for Third Sector Research, Wellington, NZ.

Fine, M.D., Graham, S. with Webb, A. (1991) *Benchmarks and other approaches to planning community support services: A review of international experience*, SPRC Reports and Proceedings 94, Sydney: Social Policy Research Centre.

Fine, M.D. and Stevens, J. (1998) 'From inmates to consumers: developments in Australian aged care since white settlement', in B. Jeawoddy and C. Saw (eds) *Successful ageing: Perspectives on health and social construction*, Sydney: Mosby.

Fine, M.D., Turvey, K. and Doyle, J. (1997) *The provision of post-hospitalisation services. Final Report*, Sydney: Social Policy Research Centre.

Fyns Stiftidende (1997a) 'God økonomi på lånt tid', 17 August, p 3.

Fyns Stiftidende (1997b) 'De har slidt og slæbt...', 4 August, p 7.

Geiser, M. and Rosendahl, B. (1995) 'Vernetzung in Altenpolitik und Altenarbeit – Begriffsklärungen und Ansätze aus der Praxis', in G. Bäcker, R. Heinze and G. Naegele (eds) *Die sozialen Dienste vor neuen Herausforderungen*, Münster: Lit, pp 148-72.

Glendinning, C. (1994) *Developing community care services for older people in Stockport: The views of service providers,* Manchester: Applied Research Centre, Department of Social Policy and Social Work, University of Manchester.

Glendinning, C. and McLaughlin, E. (1993a) *Paying for care: Lessons from Europe,* Social Security Advisory Committee Research Report 5, London: HMSO.

Glendinning, C. and McLaughlin, E. (1993b) 'Paying for informal care: lessons from Finland', *Journal of European Social Policy,* vol 3, no 4, pp 239-53.

Glendinning, C. and Rummery K. (1998) 'From collaboration to commissioning: developing relationships between general practice and social services departments', *British Medical Journal,* vol 317, pp 122-5.

Görres, S. (1992) *Geriatrische Rehabilitation und Lebensbewältigung,* Weinheim und München: Juventa.

Görres, S. (1996) 'Gesundheit und Krankheit im Alter. Defizite und Perspektiven in der Versorgungsforschung', *Zeitschrift für Gerontologie und Geriatrie,* vol 29, pp 375-81.

Grant, C. and Lapsley, H.M. (1993) *The Australian health care system 1992,* Australian Studies in Health Service Administration No 75, School of Health Services Management, Sydney: University of New South Wales.

Hamnett, C. (1995) *Inheritance in Britain: The boom that never happened,* London: PPP Lifetime plc.

Hancock, R. and Weir, P. (1994) *More ways than means: A guide to pensioners' incomes in Great Britain during the 1980s,* London: Age Concern Institute of Gerontology.

Hanninen, S., Iivari, J. and Lehto, J. (1995) *Hallittu Muutos Sosiaali ja Terveyden Huollossa?,* Jyvaskyla: Stakes, Raportteja 182, Gummerus Kirjapaino Oy.

Hansen, F. (1993) *Dynamisk geriatri. Et års erfaringer med et geriatrisk team og subakut afsnit på amtssygehuset i Glostrup,* Copenhagen: Københavns Amt.

Hansen, F., Spedtsberg, K. and Schroll, M. (1994) 'Opfølgende hjemmebesøg til ældre efter hospitals indlæggelse', *Ugeskrift for Læger,* vol 156, no 22, pp 3305-10.

Harding, T., Meredith, B. and Wistow, G. (1996) *Options for long-term care*, London: HMSO.

HC (Health Committee) (1995) *Long-term care: NHS responsibilities for meeting continuing health care needs*, House of Commons Health Committee, First Report 1995-96, vol 1, London: HMSO.

Hegner, F. (1991) 'Welche Mischung von Staat, Markt und Selbsthilfe ist die Richtige?', in M. Lewkowcez (ed) *Neues Denken in der Sozialen Arbeit: Mehr Ökologie – mehr Markt - mehr Management*, Freiburg: Lambertus, pp 121-42.

Heikkila, M. (1995) *Hyvinvoinnin paatepysakilla?*, Jyvaskyla: Stakes, Gummerus Kirjapaino Oy.

Hendriksen, C. and Strømgård, E. (1989) 'Samarbejde om gamle menneskers sygehusindlæggelse of udskrivelse, 2: Forløbet et år efter udskrivelsen', *Ugeskrift for Læger*, vol 151, no 24 pp 1534-6.

Hendriksen, C., Strømgård, E. and Sørensen, K. (1989) 'Samarbejde of gamle menneskers sygehusindlæggelse og -udskrivelse, 1: Hjemmesygeplejeskens koordinerende indsats på sygehuset', *Ugeskrift for Læger*, vol 151, no 24, pp 1531-4.

Henry Cox, R. (1998) 'The consequences of welfare reform: how conceptions of social rights are changing', *Journal of Social Policy*, vol 27, no 1, pp 1-16.

Hennessy, P. (1997) 'The growing risk of dependency in old age: what role for families and for social security?', *International Social Security Review*, vol 50, no 1, pp 23-39.

Henwood, M., Lewis, H. and Waddington, E. (1998) *Listening to users of domiciliary care services*, Brighton: Pavilion Publishing.

Hilmer, F.G. (1993) *National competition policy*, Independent Committee of Enquiry, Canberra: AGPS.

Hindle, D. and Gillett, S. (1993) *Seamless health care for the elderly: Finding a role for casemix*, University of Wollongong.

HMSO (Her Majesty's Stationery Office) (1997) *A new partnership for care in old age*, Cm 3563, London: HMSO.

Howe, A. (1996) *Interaction between acute health care and long term care: Recent developments in Australia*, Draft Report prepared for the OECD Faculty of Health Sciences, Melbourne: La Trobe University.

Hudson, B. (1998) 'Circumstances change cases: local government and the NHS', *Social Policy and Administration*, vol 32, no 1, pp 71-80.

Hugman, R. (1996) 'Health and welfare policy and older people in Europe', *Health Care in Later Life*, vol 1, no 4, pp 211-22.

Hutten, J. and Kerkstra, A. (1996) *Home care in Europe*, Aldershot: Arena.

Igl, G. (1996) 'Zum Stand der Dinge: Die Pflegeversicherung kurz vor Einführung der zweiten Stufe – Versuch einer sozialpolitischen Zwischenbewertung', *Zeitschrift für Gerontologie und Geriatrie*, no 29, pp 159-62.

Iivari, J. (1995) 'Pihavahdista portinvartijaksi', in S. Hanninen, J. Iivari and J Lehto (eds) *Hallittu Muutos Sosiaali ja Terveyden Huollossa?*, Jyvaskyla: Stakes, Raportteja 182, Gummerus Kirjapaino Oy.

Jamieson, A. (1989) 'A new age for older people? Policy shifts in health and social care', *Social Science Medicine*, vol 29, no 3, pp 445-54.

Jamieson, A. (1993) *Home care for older people in Europe: A comparison of policies and practices*, Oxford: Oxford University Press.

Jespersen, K. (1997) 'Kommunale ældreråd – en ministers tanker', *AKF Nyt* (electronic version – downloaded from http://www.akf.dk [21 November 1997]).

Jonas, I. (1996) 'Große Unterschiede bei den Einstufungen', *Pro Alter*, vol 2, p 11.

Joseph Rowntree Foundation (1996) *Meeting the costs of continuing care: Repair and recommendations*, York: Joseph Rowntree Foundation.

Jyllands-Posten (1997) 'Velfærd på aktier', 27 August, p 4.

Karjalainen, T. (1994) *Valma*, Jyvaskyla: Stakes, Raportteja 140, Gummerus Kirjapaino Oy.

Kasap and Associates (1993) *Report on the effects of the Medicare Incentive Package (MIP) on the public hospital system*, Canberra: Commonwealth Department of Health, Housing and Community Services.

KDA (1997) 'Time requirements for the care of older people', *GeroCare Newsletter 6* [Online]. Available: http://www.kda.de/gerocare/gc6e/inhalt-e.htm [1998, 20 February].

KDA (1998) 'KDA fordert mehr Geld für bessere Pflege', *Kuratorium Deutsche Altershilfe Pressemitteilung* [Online]. Available: http://www.kda.de/presse/pm110298-2.htm [1998, 20 February].

Kirk, S. and Glendinning, C. (1998) 'Trends in community care and patient participation: implications for the roles of informal carers and community nurses in the United Kingdom', *Journal of Advanced Nursing*, vol 28, no 2, pp 370-81.

Klie, T. (1995) *Pflegeversicherung*, Hannover: Vincentz.

Kock-Nielsen, I. and Nørregård, C. (1992) *Copenhagen's home care services and its users – satisfaction and confidence?*, Copenhagen: Københavns Kommune.

Koedoot, N., Hommel, A. and Knipscheer, C. (1991) *Het project Individuele Zorgsubsidie voor ouderen te Rotterdam (Evaluation of The Individual Care Subsidy Project in the Municipality of Rotterdam)*, Amsterdam: Vrije Universiteit.

Kraan, R.J., Baldock, J., Davies, B., Evers, A., Johansson, L., Knapen, M., Thorslund, M. and Tunissen, C. (1991) *Care for the elderly: Significant innovations in three European countries*, Boulder, Colorado: Westview Press.

Kroger, T. (1997) 'Local government in Scandinavia: autonomous or integrated into the welfare state?', in J. Sipilä (ed) *Social care services: The key to the Scandinavian welfare model*, Aldershot: Avebury, pp 95-108.

Laing, W. (1993) *Financing long-term care: The crucial debate*, London: Age Concern.

Landenberger, M. (1995) 'Pflegeversicherung – Modell für sozialstaatlichen Wandel', *Gegenwartskunde*, no 1, pp 19-31.

Larsen, B. (1993) *Own home as long as possible – care of the elderly – 24-hour home care service – joint operation. Primary health care in Denmark*, Copenhagen: The Danish Nurses' Organisation.

Leat, D. (1993) *The development of community care by the independent sector*, London: Policy Studies Institute.

Leeson, G.W. (1992) 'The situation of the elderly in Denmark'. *Danish Medical Bulletin*, vol 39, pp 220-3.

Leeson, G.W. (1997) *Social policy and services for older people in Denmark – the experience of DaneAge*, Paper prepared for Colloque Europèen, University of Provence, Marseilles, June 16-17.

Lehto, J. and Vaarama, M. (1996) 'Vanhuspalvelujen rakennemuutos 1988-1994', in R. Viialainen and J. Lehto (eds) *Sosiaali- ja terveyspalvelujen rakennemuutos*, Jyvaskyla: Stakes, Raportteja 192, Gummerus Kirjapaino Oy.

Lewinter, M. (1997a) 'Hjemmehjælp of hjemmehjælper i forandringens arena: spændingsfeltet mellem omsorg og effektivitet', *Kvinder, Køn og Forskning*, no 2, pp 66-77.

Lewinter, M. (1997b) *Home helps' work situation and relationship to elderly*, Paper presented to World Congress on Gerontolgy, Adelaide, Australia 19-23 August.

Lewinter, M. (1997c) 'Omsorgens puslespil', *Gerontology of samfund*, vol 13, pp 12-14.

Lewinter, M. (in preparation) *Spreading the burden of gratitude: Elderly between family and state*, University of Copenhagen, Department of Sociology.

Lewinter, M. (in press) *Home help care for elderly in Denmark: Perspectives from elderly, their family and their home helper*, Gothenburg, Sweden: Nordic School of Public Health.

Lewis, J. and Glennerster, H. (1996) *Implementing the new community care*, Buckingham: Open University Press.

LGMB (Local Government Management Board) (1997) *Community care trends 1997 report*, London: LGMB.

Lincoln Gerontology Centre Aged Care Group (1996) *Aged care system study, Victorian transition care packages report*, vol 3, Melbourne: La Trobe University.

Lorenz, W. (1994) 'Personal social services', in J. Clasen and R. Freeman (eds) *Social policy in Germany*, New York: Harvester Wheatsheaf, pp 148-69.

McCallum, J., Simons, L., Simons, J. and Wilson, J. (1994) *Hospital and home: A longitudinal study of hospital residential and community service use by older people living in Dubbo, NSW*, Best Practice paper 6, Sydney: Office on Ageing, Social Policy Directorate.

McLeay, L. (1982) *In a home or at home: Accommodation and home care for the aged*, Report of the House of Representatives Standing Committee on Expenditure, Canberra: AGPS.

Maddox, G. (1996) *Casemix classification in domiciliary nursing*, vol 2, Melbourne: Royal District Nursing Association.

Magennis, T., Oakeshott, R., Rothwell, J., Smith, D. and Truman, G. (1994) 'Sub-acute casemix: some funding implications', *Australian Casemix Bulletin*, vol 6, no 1, pp 14–16.

Makela, M. (1996) 'The organisation of primary care in Finland', in J. Griffin (ed) *The future of primary care*, London: Office of Health Economics, pp 37–45.

Meacher, M. (1972) *Taken for a ride,* London: Longman.

Melin, T. (1995) *Vanhuspalvelujen Taloudellisuus*, Saarijarvi: Stakes, Tutkimuksia 6, Gummerus Kirjapaino Oy.

Miltenburg, T. and Ramakers, C. (1996a) *Evaluatie subsidieregeling persoonsgebonden budget verpleging en verzorging 1995*, Nijmegen: Institute for Applied Social Sciences (ITS).

Miltenburg, T. and Ramakers, C. (1996b) *Voortgangsrapportage persoonsgebonden budget verpleging en verzorging verstandelijk gehandicapten 1996*, Nijmegen: Institute for Applied Social Sciences (ITS).

Ministry of Finance (1995) *Pensionssystemet og fremtidens forsørgerbyrde*, Copenhagen: Schultz.

Ministry of Interior/Home Affairs (1997) *Erfaringer med udlicitering i kommuner og amter*, Rapport udarbejdet af PLS Consult A/S, Copenhagen (electronic publication, version 1.0 downloaded from http:/www.inm.dk).

Ministry of Social Affairs (1991) *Rapport om udviklingen i hjemmeplejen*, Copenhagen.

Ministry of Social Affairs and Health (1993) *Vanhuuspolitiikkaa vuoteen 2001*, Helsinki: Edita.

Ministry of Trade and Industry, Ministry of Finance, Frederiksberg Municipality, National Association of Municipalities, Copenhagen Municipality and Ministry of Economic Affairs (1995) *Budget analyse om hjemmeplejen*, Copenhagen.

Mitchell, J., Cuthbert, M., Porter, M. and Abbott, M. (1993) 'A quality partnership: closing the gaps between hospital and the community', *Australian Clinical Review*, vol 13, no 1, pp 39-50.

Morris, A. (1994) *Home but not alone. Final Report of The House of Representatives Standing Committee on Social Affairs Enquiry into the Home and Community Care Program*, Canberra: AGPS.

Naegele, G. and Igl, G. (1993) 'Neue Aspekte in der Pflege?', *Soziale Sicherheit*, vols 8-9, pp 236-43.

National Association of Municipalities (KL) (1997) *Kommunestyret i Danmark*, Copenhagen (electronic versions downloaded from: http://www.kl.dk/kommidk/index.shtml).

NCC (National Consumer Council) (1995) *Charging consumers for services*, London: NCC.

New South Wales Aged Care Assessment Program (1996) *Evaluation Unit Report,* Department of Geriatric Medicine, Westmead Hospital.

NHS (National Health Strategy) (1991) *The Australian health jigsaw. Integration of health care delivery. Issues Paper No 1*, Canberra: AGPS.

NWECP (North West Elderly Care Project) (1996) *Managing the community care market*, Regional Analysis and Commentary, Tameside Metropolitan Borough: Department of Social Services.

Odense Kommune (1995) *Brugerundersøgelse 1995. Hjemmehjælp og plejehjem*, Samlede rapporter fra Odense Kommune, Odense: Pleje og Omsorgsafdelingen.

O'Grady, S., Fairbrother, G. and Farrington, C. (1997) 'Matching needs to services: the quick response', *Australian Health Review*, vol 19, no 4, pp 100-12.

OHE (Office of Health Economics) (1997) *Compendium of Health Statistics, 10th Edition*, London: OHE.

ONS (Office for National Statistics) (1997) *Social Trends 27*, London: HMSO.

OPCS (Office of Population Censuses and Surveys) (1995) *Subnational population projections (England)*, Series PP3, no 9, Government Statistical Service, London: HMSO.

Osborne, D. and Gaebler, T. (1992) *Reinventing government*, Reading, MA: Addison-Wesley.

Palmer, G. and Short, S. (1994) *Health care and public policy. An Australian analysis*, 2nd edn, South Melbourne: Macmillan.

Parker, R.A. (1987) *The elderly and residential care. Australian lessons for Britain*, Aldershot: Gower.

Perkins, E. and Allen, I. (1997) *Creating partnerships in social care*, London: Policy Studies Institute.

Petersen, M.D. and White, D.L. (1989) *Health care of the elderly: An information sourcebook*, Newbury Park, CA/London: Sage.

PIB (Presse- und Informationsamt der Bundesregierung) (1995) 'Pflegeversicherung – Die aktuelle Antrags- und Begutachtungssituation (309/1995)', *Sozialpolitische Umschau*, Bonn: PIB.

PIB (1996) 'Stichtag 1. Juli 1996: Start für Stationäre Pflege (209/1996)', *Sozialpolitische Umschau,* Bonn: PIB.

Plant, R. (1992) 'Citizenship, rights and welfare', in A. Coote (ed) *The welfare of citizens*, London: IPPR.

Platz, M. (1992a) *Kommunernes ældrepolitik: Fra plejehjem til egne hjem*, Copenhagen: Danish National Institute for Social Research (SFI).

Platz, M. (1992b) 'Special dwellings for the elderly', *Danish Medical Bulletin*, vol 39, no 3, pp 241-4.

Platz, M. and Petersen, N.F. (1992) *Social and economic policies and older people in Denmark*, Report for EC Actions on Older People, Copenhagen: Danish National Institute of Social Research (SFI).

Plovsing, J. (1992) *Home care in Denmark*, Copenhagen: Danish National Institute of Social Research (SFI).

Prior, D., Stewart, J. and Walsh, K. (1995) *Citizenship: Rights, community and participation*, London: Pitman.

Raassina, A. (1994) *Vanhuspolitiikka*, Helsinki: Sosiaali ja Terveysmunisterion Julkaisuja.

Ramakers, C. and Miltenburg, T. (1993) *Budget- en naturacliënten vergeleken. Experiment Cliëntgebonden Budget, Verzorging & Verpleging, III*, Nijmegen: Institute for Applied Social Sciences (ITS).

Ramakers, C. and Miltenburg, T. (1997) *Voortgangsrapportage persoongebonden budget verpleging en verzorging verstandelijk gehandicapten 1997*, Nijmegen: Institute for Applied Social Sciences (ITS).

Rasmussen, E.T. (1997) *Ældreprojektet – en evaluaering, Arbejdspapir*, Copenhagen: Danish National Institute of Social Research (SFI).

Richards, E., Wilsdon, T. and Lyons, S. (1996) *Paying for long-term care*, London: Institute for Public Policy Research.

Robinson, J. and Turnock, S. (1998) *Investing in rehabilitation*, London: King's Fund and The Audit Commission.

Robinson, R. and Steiner, A. (1998) *Managed health care*, Buckingham: Open University Press.

Rold Andersen, B. (1993) 'Dansk ældrepolitik', *Fremtidens ældrepolitik*, Lundbeckfondens prisopgave 1992, Copenhagen: Jurrist- og Økonomforbundets Forlag.

Romijn, C., Coolen, J., de Klerk, M., Koedoot, C., van Linschoten, C., Perenboom, M. and Ruisen, R. (1991) *Demonstratieprojecten in de ouderenzorg (Demonstrating Innovations in Long-Term Care for Elderly People)*, Nijmegen: Institute for Applied Social Sciences (ITS).

Rønnow, B. (1996) *Tillægsydelser i velfærdsservicen*, Copenhagen: Danish National Institute of Social Research (SFI).

Rummery, K. and Glendinning, C. (1997a) *Working together: Primary care involvement in commissioning social care services*, Debates in Primary Care No 2, Manchester: NPCRDC.

Rummery, K. and Glendinning, C. (1997b) *Negotiating needs, access and gatekeeping*, Paper given to conference on 'Citizenship and the Welfare State: Fifty Years of Progress', Ruskin College, Oxford, December.

Salter, B. (1994) 'The politics of community care: social rights and welfare limits', *Policy and Politics*, vol 22, pp 117-31.

Saper, R. and Laing, W. (1995) 'Age of uncertainty', *Health Services Journal*, 26 October.

Saunders, P. and Fine, M.D. (1992) 'The mixed economy of support for the aged in Australia. Lessons for privatisation', *The Economic and Labour Relations Review*, vol 3, no 2, pp 18-42.

Sax, S. (1984) *A strife of interests. Politics and policies in Australian health services*, Sydney: George Allen and Unwin.

Schmidt, M. (1988) *Sozialpolitik*, Opladen: Leske & Budrich.

Schneekloth, U. (1996) 'Entwicklung von Pflegebedürftigkeit im Alter', *Zeitschrift für Gerontologie und Geriatrie*, vol 29, pp 11-17.

Scotton, D. (1995) 'Managed competition: issues for Australia', *Australian Health Review*, vol 17, no 3, pp 82-104.

Sejr, T., Eskelinen, L. and Boll Hansen, E. (1995) 'Ældre i behandlingssystmet', *AKF Nyt*, vol 1(marts), pp 2-9.

Senate Select Committee (1984) *Private nursing homes in Australia: Their conduct, administration and ownership*, Report by Senate Select Committee on Private Hospitals and Nursing Homes, Canberra: AGPS.

Sipilä, J. (1997) *Social care services: The key to the Scandinavian welfare model*, Aldershot: Avebury.

Sipilä, J. and Anttonen, A. (1994) 'Payments for care in Finland', in A. Evers, M. Pijl and C. Ungerson (eds) *Payments for care*, Aldershot: Avebury and Vienna: European Centre.

Sociaal en Cultureel Planbureau (1997) *Vraagverkenning wonen en zorg voor ouderen*, Rijswijk.

Stathers, G.M. and Gonski, P.N. (1996) 'Outcome of attendance by an elderly population to an emergency department, as measured by a behavioural model', *Australian Journal on Ageing*, vol 15, no 1, pp 38-41.

Stratmann, J. and Korte, E. (1993) 'Aspekte der Entwicklung von Bedarfsrichtwerten für soziale Dienste und Einrichtungen der örtlichen Altenarbeit und ihrer kleinräumigen Planung', in S. Kühnert and G. Naegele (eds) *Perspektiven moderner Altenpolitik und Altenarbeit*, Hannover: Vincentz, pp 197-216.

Street, P. (1995) *Post-acute community services study*, Melbourne: Bundoora Centre for Applied Gerontology and Preston and Northcote Community Hospital.

Swane, C.E. (1994) 'Payments for care: the case of Denmark', in A. Evers, M. Pijl and C. Ungerson (eds) *Payments for care: A comparative overview*, Aldershot: Avebury.

Sykes, R. and Leather, P. (1997) *Grey matters: A survey of older people in England*, Anchor Research.

Tatchell, M. (1983) 'Measuring hospital output: a review of the service mix and case mix approaches', *Social Science and Medicine*, vol 17, no 13, pp 871-83.

Tester, S. (1996) *Community care for older people: A comparative perspective*, Basingstoke: Macmillan.

Thornton, P. and Tozer, R. (1995) *Having a say in change: Older people and community care*, York: Joseph Rowntree Foundation.

Tilia, G.B. (1995) *Helse og hjemmeservice i Esbjerg Kommune. En brugerundersøgelse af den integrerede hjemmepleje*, Esbjerg: Sydjysk Universitetscenter. Institut for Samfunds- og erhvervsudvikling, Notat 22/95.

Townsend, P. (1963) *The last refuge*, London: Routledge.

TCP (Transition Care Program) National (1996) *National evaluation*, Canberra: Department of Human Services and Health.

Udviklingskontoret (1994) *Brugerundersøgelse af hjemmehjælpen*, Århus: Århus Municipality.

Uusitalo, H. (1996) *Economic crisis and social policy in Finland in the 1990s*, Discussion Paper No 70, Sydney: University of New South Wales, Social Policy Research Centre.

Vaarama, M. (1995) *Vanhusten Hoivapalvelujen tuloksellisuus Hyvinvoinnin Tuotanto-Nakokulmasta*, Jyvaskyla: Stakes, Tutkimuksia 55, Gummerus Kirjapaino Oy.

Vaarama, M. and Hurskanen, R. (1993) *Vanhuspolitiikan Tulevaisuus Kuvat ja Kehittamisstrategiat*, Jyvaskyla: Stakes, Gummerus Kirjapaino Oy.

Viialainen, R. and Lehto, J. (1996) *Sosiaali ja Terveyspalvelujen Rakennemuutos*, Jyvaskyla: Stakes, Raportteja 140, Gummerus Kirjapaino Oy.

Wagner, L. (1989) 'A proposed model for care of the elderly', *International Nursing Review*, vol 36, no 2, pp 50-3, 60.

Wagner, L. (1992) 'Non-institutional care for the elderly. A Danish model', *Danish Medical Bulletin*, vol 39, no 3, pp 236-8.

Wagner, L. (1994) *Innovations in primary health care for elderly people in Denmark. Two action research projects*, Doctoral Thesis, Gothenburg: The Nordic School of Public Health.

Wagner, L. (1995) 'Indførelsen af nye methoder i pleje og omsorg af ældre i Danmark', *Tidskrift for Sygeplejeforskning*, vol 2, no 11, pp 25-37.

Wagner, L. (1997) 'Long-term care in the Danish health care system', *Health Care Management: State of the Art Reviews*, June, pp 149-56.

Walker, A. (1994) *Half a century of promises: The failure to realise 'community care' for older people*, London: The 1994 Graham Lecture, National Westminster Hall.

Walker, A. (1995) 'Integrating the family into a mixed economy of care', in I. Allen and E. Perkins (eds) *The future of family care for older people*, London: HMSO.

Walker, A. and Maltby, T. (1997) *Ageing Europe*, Buckingham: Open University Press.

Weekers, S. and Pijl. M. (1998) *Home care and care allowances in the European Union*, Utrecht: Netherlands Institute of Care and Welfare.

Wilson, G. (1994) 'Assembling their own care packages: payments for care by men and women in advanced old age', *Health and Social Care in the Community*, vol 2, no 5, pp 283-91.

Winters, S. (1991) 'Verteilungswirkungen einer Gesetzlichen Pflegeversicherung: eine Replik', *Wirtschaftsdienst*, vol IX, pp 478-80.

Wistow, G. (1996) 'The changing scene in Britain', in T. Harding, B. Meredith and G. Wistow (eds) *Options for long-term care*, London: HMSO.

Wistow, G., Knapp, M., Hardy, B., Forder, J., Kendall, J. and Manning, R. (1996) *Social care markets: Progress and prospects*, Buckingham: Open University Press.

Ziekenfondsraad (1995) *Regeling Ziekenfondsraad subsidiëring zorgvernieuwing, verpleging en verzorging 1995,* Amstelveen, no 661.

Zijderveld-Blom, A. and Coolen, J. (1992) *Experiment beschermd wonen met flexibel zorgaanbod (Experiments with very sheltered housing),* Enschede: Universiteit Twente/Centrum voor Bestuurskundig Onderzoek.

Index